Men's Health

This comprehensive book addresses men's health and wellness in the context of the male psyche, provides up to date research on men's health, discusses theoretical frameworks, shares perspectives from men and lists consumer resources and tools.

Men's Health explores social, cultural, physical and psychological approaches to men's health with sections focusing on the psycho-social issues, the body, relationships, healthy living and aging, while taking into account cultural differences. Each chapter:

- provides a review of the current science and emerging research of the topic;
- outlines theoretical frameworks, best practices and recommendations for advancing men's health through service delivery, research, education, policy and advocacy;
- features a personal assessment tool on the topic; and
- includes vignettes from men, their friends and families, and care providers.

Suitable for students taking undergraduate courses on men's health and wellness, this broad-ranging textbook is the ideal introduction to the topic.

Diana Karczmarczyk is a Master Certified Health Education Specialist who holds an MPH degree in public health with a focus on community health education and a PhD in Education with a minor in public health and a specialization in international education. She has been teaching public health courses in higher education for almost 20 years on topics including men's health, sexuality and human behavior, health education and promotion, health behavior theory, program planning and evaluation, personal health and wellness, social determinants of health, and community needs assessments and partnerships.

Susan A. Milstein is a Master Certified Health Education Specialist and a Certified Sexuality Educator. She has an MA in Health Education and a PhD in Human Sexuality Education. Dr. Milstein is a clinical assistant professor in the Department of Health and Kinesiology at Texas A & M University. She is the Continuing Education Coordinator for the Woodhull Freedom Foundation, a member of the Advisory Board for the Men's Health Network, and a member of the Advisory Board for the *American Journal of Sexuality Education*.

Men's Health

An Introduction

**Edited by Diana Karczmarczyk
and Susan A. Milstein**

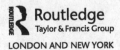
Routledge
Taylor & Francis Group

LONDON AND NEW YORK

First published 2021
by Routledge
2 Park Square, Milton Park, Abingdon, Oxon OX14 4RN

and by Routledge
605 Third Avenue, New York, NY 10017

Routledge is an imprint of the Taylor & Francis Group, an informa business

British Library Cataloguing-in-Publication Data
A catalogue record for this book is available from the British Library

Library of Congress Cataloging-in-Publication Data
Names: Karczmarczyk, Diana, editor. | Milstein, Susan A., editor.
Title: Men's health : an introduction / edited by
Diana Karczmarczyk and Susan A. Milstein.
Description: Abingdon, Oxon ; New York, NY : Routledge, 2020. |
Includes bibliographical references and index.
Identifiers: LCCN 2020008350 (print) | LCCN 2020008351 (ebook) |
ISBN 9781138496057 (hardback) | ISBN 9781138496064 (paperback) |
ISBN 9781351022620 (ebook)
Subjects: LCSH: Men–Health and hygiene.
Classification: LCC RA777.8 .M462 2020 (print) |
LCC RA777.8 (ebook) | DDC 613/.0423–dc23
LC record available at https://lccn.loc.gov/2020008350
LC ebook record available at https://lccn.loc.gov/2020008351

ISBN: 978-1-138-49605-7 (hbk)
ISBN: 978-1-138-49606-4 (pbk)
ISBN: 978-1-351-02262-0 (ebk)

Typeset in Bembo
by Newgen Publishing UK

Visit the eResources: www.routledge.com/9781138496064

Dedicated to Dr. David Anderson.
Because of your constant support and incredible mentorship, this book happened. Thank you for always believing in me and in this idea, supporting and challenging me to pursue my passion, and reminding me that I can make an important contribution in the world.

Diana Karczmarczyk PhD, MPH, MCHES

Contents

Figures

Tables

Contributors

Adam E. Barry is a health behavior social scientist, with specific training and expertise in alcohol use, alcohol-induced impairment, and intoxication. Barry's research spans the assessment and measurement of alcohol-related behaviors, impaired driving and intoxication, and protective behavioral strategies to minimize intoxication. Barry's work has garnered national and international attention. He has been a featured guest on prominent television news programs in the United States, such as CNN, as well as the Canadian national news program CTV. Online and print media outlets such as the *New York Times, The Atlantic, Los Angeles Times,* and NBC News have also featured his work.

Armin Brott has, over the past 20 years, helped shape perceptions of fathers and the vital role they play in their children's lives. Hailed by *Time Magazine* as "the superdad's superdad," Armin is passionate about improving the health and wellbeing of men, at any age. He is the author of *Blueprint for Men's Health, Your Head: An Owner's Manual* and has contributed to *The New York Times Magazine, Newsweek, American Baby, Parenting, Child, Men's Health, The Washington Post* and other major publications. Armin is on the Board of Advisors of Men's Health Network and the founder of MrDad.com.

Emil T. Chuck began his research career after earning his degree in Cell Biology from Case Western Reserve University, focusing his work on cardiac electrophysiology. His postdoctoral research looked at mechanisms of heart failure and sudden cardiac death. His research awards include fellowships from the Heart Rhythm Society and the Novartis Foundation. While his career has focused more on higher education administration, he continues to read and review clinical trials focused on cardiovascular device development.

Norman Eburne graduated from the University of Oregon in Health Education with cognate areas in endocrinology and reproductive physiology. His dissertation focused on psychiatric education research and training. His assignments have included developing drug information and rehabilitation centers, editing professional journals, boards of directors of health organizations, contributing to several books and other publications, rural family health specialist for the USDA, developing programs in school and community health. While working with young men regarding masculine roles, he gained insight concerning the male mode of thinking and how it relates to seeking of health care.

Sara K. Fehr is a Clinical Assistant Professor in the Department of Health and Kinesiology at Texas A&M University. She earned her PhD in Health Education from the University of Cincinnati with a cognate emphasis in women's health and human sexuality. Her research interests include the prevention of STIs, unplanned pregnancies, and intimate partner violence. Dr. Fehr is a certified facilitator for the Green Dot and STAND Up programs, which work to reduce power-based personal violence on campuses. She is also a certified sexual assault survivor advocate and works as a volunteer for the local sexual assault resource center.

Salvatore J. Giorgianni, Jr. is the Principle Founding Partner of Griffon Consulting Group, Inc. He is the author of over 70 peer-reviewed and general publications in men's health, health policy and pharmacotherapy. He is one of the Founders and Chair-Emeritus of the American Public Health Association's Men's Health caucus. He is Senior Science Adviser and spokesperson for the Men's Health Network. He previously held a series of executive positions at Pfizer, Inc. He has worked on development and medical-marketing programs for numerous multibillion-dollar pharmaceuticals including Zithromax, Zoloft, Aricept and Viagra.

Courtney M. Gonzalez received her BS degree in Global and Community Health from George Mason University. She joined Inova Health as a clinical technician in 2017 and holds a certificate as a health education specialist (CHES). She is also the co-founder of Weske & Company, a health education company focused on inclusive health education. In November 2016, she published her first research article, 'Sex Education Policy: Need for a Standard Definition of Medically Accurate Information' in the journal *Pedagogy in Health Promotion*. She is the co-author of *It's GREAT to be YOU!*, a children's book that promotes diversity.

Stephen Howes received his MEd in education from Lamar University and a BSEd in Health & Physical Education from George Mason University. He currently serves as an Adjunct Professor of Health at George Mason University and has over ten years of teaching experience in Fairfax County Public Schools teaching secondary Health & Physical Education.

Zachary A. Jackson received his PhD in Health Education from Texas A&M University. His research focuses on social factors (i.e., discrimination and sense of belonging) that impact college students' educational performance and their health. Dr. Jackson is also interested in investigating how these social factors differ among students based on the type of institution they attend. His work raises awareness about the influence of gender and culture on health outcomes and provides health education and social support to boys and men of color.

James E. Leone is a Professor of Public Health at Bridgewater State University. Dr. Leone previously held faculty appointments at The George Washington University, Northeastern University, and Southern Illinois University. He has published numerous peer-reviewed articles and presented his research over 200 times in a variety of research conferences and symposia. Dr. Leone's academic interests include: male health, body image, drug abuse epidemiology, celiac disease and issues in professional development. He has written chapters for various textbooks, and authored a book on male health entitled *Concepts in Male Heath: Perspectives across the Lifespan*.

Razan Maxson is a University of Central Florida graduate who has worked with Dr. Michael J. Rovito since 2017 in the field of men's health research and men's behavioral health research. As a research coordinator for the Behavioral Health Research Group (BHRG) Razan has helped to lead and mentor others in Dr. Rovito's methods of research and publication. He has also worked in developing new methods for sex education at a collegiate level and is an advocate for the betterment of sexual education for all.

Kayla K. McDonald is an Adjunct Professor within the Department of Global and Community Health at George Mason University, where she received her Bachelor of Science in Community Health and Master of Public Health with a concentration on community health promotion. Kayla is an administrative assistant for the Arc of Greater Prince William/INSIGHT, where she assists in the planning, implementation and evaluation of services provided by Family Support Services, in addition to special projects. Her interests include youth development, physical activity and the intersectionality of social determinants of health.

Katie Potestio joined Capital District Physicians' Health Plan (CDPHP) in 2016 as a population health and wellness specialist in the population health and wellness department. In her role, she works on projects related to maternal and preventive health, nutrition and worksite wellness. Prior to CDPHP, Katie supported state public health department chronic disease prevention efforts with the Association of State and Territorial Health Officials. She earned a Bachelor's degree in Biology from Haverford College outside Philadelphia and a Master's degree in Public Health from the University of Washington in Seattle. Katie is a registered dietitian, mother of two children and an outdoor enthusiast.

Michael J. Rovito is an Assistant Professor of Health Sciences at the University of Central Florida and a certified health education specialist. He holds a PhD in Public Health and an MA in Urban Studies from Temple University and a BA in Geography from Millersville University. His work specializes in testicular self-examination and testicular cancer, male health behavioral change, instrumentation design and health communication. Dr. Rovito is the Founder/Chairman of The Male Wellness Collective.

Alex M. Russell is a Doctoral Candidate at Texas A&M University who will graduate in the spring of 2020. His research broadly focuses on alcohol use and misuse among adolescent and young adult populations. Specifically, his work has examined the following areas: (1) peer influences on college students' alcohol use, (2) alcohol marketing to youth via online and social media, and (3) the protective effects of youth religiosity/spirituality on early onset of alcohol use.

Barry Sharp, before retiring, spent more than 24 years as a health educator with the Texas Department of State Health Services, with about 18 years in leadership roles at the state and national levels in tobacco prevention and control. Other areas in public health that he worked included health promotion, community and worksite wellness and community preparedness. Prior to public health, he was a journalist at newspapers in Texas and Oklahoma. He is currently working with special education students at a local high school. He is an ordained deacon in the United Methodist Church focusing on health and marriage ministry.

Ledric D. Sherman received his PhD from Texas A&M University in August of 2013. Dr. Sherman's research interests are focused on Type 2 diabetes self-management, men's health, quality and quantity of life among people with type 2 diabetes, and health education and wellness promotion. Dr. Sherman enjoys teaching and mentoring students to help prepare them for the next chapter in their lives, both professionally and personally. Dr. Sherman has taught undergraduate courses in environmental health, grant writing, healthy lifestyles, and contemporary issues for community health interns. He also has experience in teaching program planning for graduate students.

Preface

The impetus for the book originally was as a result of me teaching human sexuality. In this course, many of the available textbooks tend to come from a female-centered, cisgender and heteronormative perspective. It is typically the story of man meets woman, there is a sperm and an egg, they have babies and live happily ever after. Classroom instruction counters that narrative as much as possible with lots of information and alternate perspectives. I found that any time there was a topic about men's health, whether it was infertility or challenges in relationships, or anything that came through a gendered lens it always caught the attention of my students. They were truly curious to learn more. Unfortunately, we did not always have either the time in the course or the data to go into the topics further. The same thing happened in other courses that I taught that included discussions on nutrition, weight management and emotional health. Many times these topics raised a lot of questions that had a lot to do with gender expectations and norms.

I was supposed to be the only editor of this book, but during the process, one of the chapter authors, Dr. Susan A. Milstein, offered to share her editing experience. Because this is a unique contribution in such an important space, having an additional editor helped me challenge my ideas and perspectives, ultimately resulting in a stronger and comprehensive finished product.

This book was always intended to be an edited work. The original idea came about because there were not many books on this topic that were coming from a health perspective. They were often psychology or sociology books. I felt like there were so many things I wanted to make sure were tackled in a book on men's health, and I knew that there were people who were working with men that could speak to specific topics. These subject matter experts would be able to identify best practices, policy recommendations, programs and efforts, and the current research. Authors were given general guidelines on what to address for each chapter. Specifically they were asked to provide information from an international perspective, and to give suggestions for books and movies for further reading and exploration. Because this is an edited work, each chapter will feel different to the reader, as every author was encouraged to use their own voice.

Each chapter also includes a story and personal assessments. Sometimes the story is from men, sometimes it is about them, but the idea is for the reader to get an idea of what men experience with regard to each topic. The personal assessments are designed to allow the reader the chance to reflect on each topic. These stories and personal assessments were designed to create a book that could serve not only as a textbook for a college course, but also as a resource for anyone in the world who cares about men's health.

Diana Karczmarczyk PhD, MPH, MCHES

Acknowledgments

We would like to thank the many individuals who helped to make this book a reality. We want to offer our thanks to the team at Routledge, especially Grace McInnes, for your complete support for this project and guiding us through all the stages to publication, even when the project fell off the track for a bit; to the contributors, thank you for sharing your expertise on these various and important topics in such thoughtful and detailed chapters; to the individuals who shared their perspectives for the "In His Own Words" sections throughout the book, thank you for trusting us with your words and sharing them with others so we can all learn and improve men's health; and, to Kayla Hense and Thomas Brunot, thank you for inspiring us with your work on exploring masculinity through the eyes of men – we appreciate your contribution in the book and wish much success for the upcoming exhibition of your work.

Part I

Male psyche

1 Introduction to men's health

Susan A. Milstein and Diana Karczmarczyk

What is health?

In order to have a discussion about men's health, it's important to first define the word "health." In decades past, being sick or healthy were seen as two sides of a coin, you were either one or the other. Looking at health this way is limiting because it does not take into account that while someone might not be sick, that doesn't mean they're healthy. Defining people as only being sick or healthy also doesn't speak to their quality of life.

Did you know?

In the preamble of its constitution, the World Health Organization defines health as "a state of complete physical, mental and social well-being and not merely the absence of disease or infirmity."

(2019a, para. 1)

In the 1980s the wellness movement became recognized worldwide, and this helped to change how we talk about health (WHO, 2019b). This movement brought with it a new way of looking at health, creating models where there were multiple dimensions of health and wellness instead of focusing solely on whether someone is sick or healthy. Today the terms health and wellness are often used interchangeably, and there are multiple models of health and wellness that exist. Most models use four similar basic dimensions of health: physical, spiritual, social and psychological, and all of these dimensions can be thought of as existing on a continuum. It's important to include a discussion of these dimensions in a book on men's health because many men equate physical health with general health, while often ignoring the other dimensions.

Physical health is how the body is functioning. Physical health is not the same as one's overall health. It's possible to have a healthy looking physique, and have high cholesterol. It's possible to be managing a long-term chronic disease, and ultimately die because of old age and not complications related to the disease.

Spiritual health is a person's understanding that their life has purpose. For some people, spiritual health is linked to their religious beliefs. Whether a person is religious or not, spiritual health is still an important component of one's overall health.

Social health is about the relationships that one forms with other people. It's important to note, especially at a time when some people focus on the number of followers they have on social media and the number of likes or views their posts get, that social health is not necessarily about the number of friends you have. Social health is about the quality of the relationships you have with others, whether they are offline or online.

In some models, emotional and mental health are separated into two distinct dimensions, but in others they are presented under the umbrella term of psychological health. Psychological health is not merely the presence or absence of mental illness. It's also about people's ability to recognize and understand emotions and the ability to express emotions in a healthy way.

Did you know?

Men are 24% less likely than women to have visited a doctor in the past 12 months.
(AHRQ, 2012)

In his own words

Ali Rezaian, George Mason University, student – class of 2016
The fact is that a majority of common health issues affecting men are not receiving the attention that they should. Much of this may simply have to do with men attempting to align with the commonly held perceptions of them in today's society, where their masculinity is seemingly compromised if they take an interest in seeking help. Statistics on health discrepancies between men and women are alarming to say the least. Men also deal with many more emotional troubles than people realize, as well.

Socio-ecological model

There are many theories about what shapes the health behaviors of individuals. The socio-ecological model (SEM) describes the different levels of influence that explain people's behaviors and who or what may impact them in changing their behaviors (Kilanowski, 2017). At the core of this model is the principle that individuals are shaped by their environment and those around them, and how individuals can impact the environment and those around them. The model is typically depicted with nested circles with the inner-most circle being the individual, referred to as intrapersonal (see Figure 1.1). Individuals have their own knowledge, beliefs and existing health behaviors. In health promotion efforts, the focus on this level usually results in directing education and/or developing the skill set of the individual to improve their health. The next circle closest to the individual is indicated by the interpersonal level of influence. This level includes the individual's friends or family. These are the people in the individual's life that can impact the choices they make about health. For example, an individual who smokes is influenced by their family members. So, if the individual wants to quit smoking but the rest of the family continues to smoke, then the likelihood of that individual being successful lowers. However, if the rest of the family members that smoke also quit, then the chances are higher that the individual will be able to successfully quit.

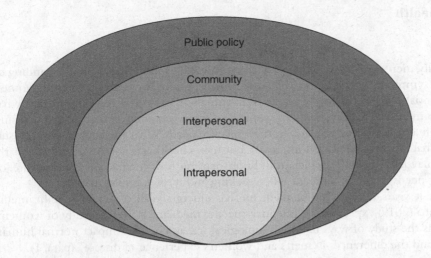

Figure 1.1 Levels of influence in the socio-ecological model.
Source: Developed by Susan A. Milstein, 2019.

The next level of influence is typically indicated as community. This can include where the individual lives, works, plays or prays. For example, if the individual works in a company that promotes physical activity and there is a soccer/football field nearby, then the individual may be more likely to join the soccer/football team and play on a regular basis. Finally, the model recognizes that policies and/or laws at the local, state and national levels can influence behavior. However, a policy alone may not change behavior. For example, there may be a law in place that drivers and all passengers in a motor vehicle wear their seat belt. Though many will use their seat belts, there is not a guarantee that all will. So, if all levels are addressed simultaneously with public health promotion efforts, then it increases the chances that an individual may learn new information or a skill, be reminded to behave in a specific way because a friend also learned new information or a skill, be reminded, or even supported, to behave in a way in their community, or follow the direction of a policy.

Using the SEM as a framework to view men's health is important. Just by reading this book it is possible that individuals may change their beliefs about men's health. It is also possible that some may change their own behaviors. If someone learns new information or develops a skill as a result of this book and shares that with another individual, then the second level of influence (interpersonal) comes into play. Ultimately, the messages that are shared throughout this book will challenge communities across the globe to consider how they support men in achieving optimal health and wellness. These philosophical shifts can then be supported with legislation.

Did you know?

Men are twice as likely as women to meet the criteria for alcohol dependence at some point in their lives.

(Hasin, Stinson, Ogburn, & Grant, 2007)

Men's health

The past

Historically, men were the focus of medical research. This meant that the understanding of signs and symptoms of disease, as well as treatment options, were male centered. Women were essentially neglected in the research. Eventually there was a recognition that what applied to men didn't always apply to women, so there was a movement toward focusing on women and dedicating research to their specific needs. What has happened as a result of this is that women's health has improved, but men's health has not. Also, while the early research may have focused on men, it did not focus on how men access medical care, or how their needs might be different when seeking and receiving information.

In recent years, a new type of medicine has emerged, called gender-specific medicine. Legato (2019) explains that "[g]ender-specific medicine is not the study of women's health; it is the study of ways in which biological sex and gender impact normal human function and the differences in men's and women's experience of disease" (para. 1).

In his own words

Anonymous, Interviewee #4, shared by Kayla Hense and Thomas Brunot

Growing up, his idea of being a father was providing food and house. That was it. We never really did father-son things, typical things like throwing a ball around. He was always working, so what I got from that was take care of your friends and family, and to me that's a masculine thing to do – being there for people financially. My mother and my older sister taught me how to be there for people emotionally. They taught me how to be a gentleman – how to treat women with respect and simple stuff like that. Everything else about how to be a man (well what my idea of what a man should be) I learned on my own.

The present

In general, when we talk about health, we're usually talking about it because things aren't going well. The truth is that there is something wrong with the health of men, and we haven't done enough to improve their health. Men are suffering more than women. While it may be that they interpret pain differently from women, the data supports that pain is negatively impacting their quality of life. Men are dying younger than women in every region of the world (Baker et al., 2014). In order to even begin addressing the health disparities between men and women, we need to address one of the biggest issues impacting men's health, which is that of masculinity.

There are many ways that masculinity can be manifested. Traditional masculinity implies that men are strong, that they feel no pain, and that they don't need help with anything. What these views have done is create generations of men and boys who feel that their need to be strong is more important than their need to take care of themselves. Traditional masculinity has taught men that it's not okay to be emotional, but that it's okay to be violent and aggressive. This directly impacts men's mental and physical health, as well as their relationships with others. If a man is taught that he doesn't feel sad or hopeless, he is not going to willingly seek out help for mental health issues. What he may do instead is turn to alcohol to mask what he's feeling, which can then impact those around him.

What this also means is that when the topic of men's health is discussed, some men may see it as an attack on their masculinity, implying that they are weak or damaged. This perceived attack may make some men feel vulnerable, embarrassed, or scared which may prevent them from seeking medical care. These feelings can also be exacerbated by the fact that many of the questions that are asked by doctors may put them on the defensive, for example, "Why didn't you do something about this sooner?" This is one of the reasons why, when men do go to the doctor, the illness or pain has progressed to a point where they have limited treatment options.

Did you know?

Men are almost four times more likely to die by suicide than women.

(Centers for Disease Control and Prevention, 2015)

In his own words

Larry Jayson, 72. Father, grandfather

In August or September of 2018 when I got out of the shower, I noted a little drop of blood on my left nipple. It happened two or three times, it was never more than a trickle, and I put on a band aid and the next day there would be no blood. The third time it happened, I called my doctor's office. I got a call from her office the next day saying "get your butt over to the cancer center and do it now." They did some tests and found cancer on the left side, and one or two spots on the right side. At the beginning of October, I had a double mastectomy. My doctor said that only 3% of cases he's ever done were on men. When it first happened I didn't feel like I wanted to talk to anyone about it. I told my board of directors and my staff, but other than those in my closest inner circle, I didn't tell anyone what was going on. Now I want people to know it's nothing to be embarrassed about. I want men to know if they see it early, if they feel if there's something wrong, it pays to catch it and to live with it. If you're embarrassed and don't know what to do about it, you take the chance that a lot worse is going to happen. The first time I walked into the cancer center, they said you have to put on a pink robe, I said "are you kidding me? I'm telling you now, there will be blue robes in this place for the guys who are coming in after me," and there are.

There are other ways that the traditional health care system does not help men feel comfortable as patients. For many men, a large part of their masculine identity is being the breadwinner of the family. This may mean that if they have to choose between seeking health care for an injury or an illness or working and earning money, they often choose working and earning money. The traditional health care system often forces men to make that choice. In addition, when men do access health care, they may find themselves in waiting rooms that are not male friendly. Many waiting rooms are open concept spaces, leaving little physical privacy, that have reading materials aimed at women, such as popular women-focused magazines.

This lack of intentionality in design for spaces also extends to scientific studies. For example, the scientific community is not consistent with the use of language in the literature. Specifically, the terms male and men are not typically defined or used consistently. As a result, throughout this book men and male are used interchangeably. In addition, while the terms sex and gender are often used interchangeably, they are not the same. Sex refers to biological differences, and while many assume that it means either a male or female, it would be more accurate to think of sex as a continuum, with male on one end, female on the other, and a variety of differentiation between. Sex will impact health based on the presence of specific hormones, chromosomes, and organs. A woman's risk of heart attack is lower than a man's prior to menopause, because of the protective factor of estrogen. This means that despite our interest in making this book inclusive of all people who identify as male or a man, most times the data was not available to indicate who was being represented in the studies.

To try to address the limited diversity of men in the data, there are real stories from men throughout the book, sharing details of their experiences. Some of these stories include very specific information such as the individual's age, where they live, their occupation, and the number of children they have, while other contributions are by men who only felt comfortable being identified as anonymous, which speaks volumes about how they experience these topics.

In his own words

Cody Roberts, 20

We continue to be shown that a man is only worth what others can take away from a glance, a male's physical embodiment is always focused on in society, what is taking place inside is cast out of sight and out of mind. When we begin to learn what is actually going on with our bodies and how we work, it is all physical, we will grow hair, our voice will get deeper, and so on. We are lectured endlessly about how our bodies will change, but are never taught how our minds react to our growth, because society doesn't seem to care. Men are loosely taught how to be respectful, how to treat a woman, how to be respectful yet also demand respect even if it involves violence, yet we are never taught how to respect ourselves. Many men aren't given a place to share their emotions, so they don't, they recede to their physical teachings, exact power over others begging for societal recognition. We are taught that men don't cry, because if you do you are weak, we are shown that our emotions are not acceptable, so we pretend they don't exist, no matter how badly it hurts.

The future

Men's health is a global issue. In 2014, the World Health Organization highlighted that there is a gap in the health of men when compared to women, and that men's health topics need to be addressed as part of strategic plans moving forward (Baker et al., 2014). In order to accomplish this, there needs to be a reframing of how we think and talk about men's health. Men's health is not merely adding the word "men" in front of a topic and thinking that there's no differentiation by gender. Around the globe, this may be done through the creation of offices of men's health to support programmatic efforts that address the needs of men at the local level This may be done at the state, province or territory level. Currently in the United States there are only 14 out of 50 states that have dedicated offices or coordinators to support efforts for men's health (Fadich, Llamas, Giorgianni, Stephenson, & Nwaiwu, 2018). Another strategy is to integrate men's health into nationwide health improvement plans. In the United Kingdom, there have been efforts made by the Men's Health Forum (n.d.) to have the government create a Men's Health Policy outlining a comprehensive approach to men's health. In the United States, however, there is no national Office on Men's Health similar to the one that exists for women. Though there have been efforts made to create such a national office for 17 years, to date it has been unsuccessful (W. K. Kellogg Foundation, 2003). This lack of equitable resources for men has been called out as a "federal indifference" of the White House by menshealth.com (The Editors of Men's Health, 2015, para. 1).

Globally, there is a critical need to identify ways to create educational campaigns that speak to men in ways that they can hear, understand, and which enable them to apply new skills to improve their health. For instance, many tend to see health care in the family as a woman's role, so much of what we do in terms of educating men about men's health is actually targeting the women in their lives. This can be an issue, since men access health care differently from women. This means that changing the way that providers interact with men as patients is key. By recognizing that when men are exposing parts of their body that hurt or may not function in their ideal way they are vulnerable, we can start to work through the confines of masculinity. Tailoring approaches to target men by breaking down barriers to encourage them to talk about their health needs and issues in a safe, trusted space is needed. In addition, offering appointment hours that don't conflict with work may make men more likely to access health care.

Despite what might seem like an enormous task and responsibility, there have been many efforts made to better address the needs of men, specifically in regard to whether or not they are accessing health care. Man Cave Health, located in New York, is designed to provide men with more comfortable surroundings. The waiting rooms are sports themed, with leather chairs and flat-screen TVs (Man Cave Health, 2018). One of the reasons for creating Man Cave Health, which currently focuses specifically on men who are at risk of prostate cancer, is the idea that if the offices feel more comfortable and less clinical, men would be more willing to go regularly (Man Cave Health, 2018). These kinds of changes to decor, in addition to having more male nurses and receptionists, can help men feel more comfortable from the moment they walk in for medical care (Banks, 2001). The concept of using sports to target men has been used in non-medical settings as well. A program in Scotland called Football Fans in Training was designed to help overweight and obese men, between the ages of 35 and 65, make healthy changes (Gray et al., 2013).

According to Northern Health (2011), Canada's efforts to address men's health formalized about 20 years ago with the Toronto Men's Health movement which focused primarily on specific health-related issues impacting men. Since then, the movement evolved to use the "go to where the men are" approach, placing programs within reach for men to access more easily (Northern Health, 2011). Northern Health released *Where are the men?*, a report on the status of men and boys in northern British Columbia (BC)

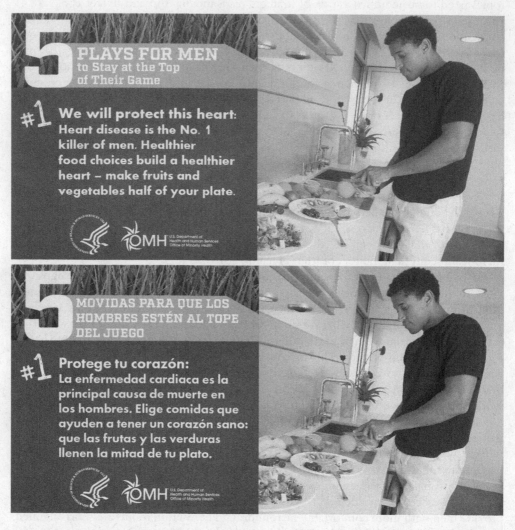

Figure 1.2 Office of Minority Health's Five Plays for Men's Health. This comparative view of
English and Spanish versions of a public service announcement used during men's health
month in the United States is one of five that promotes healthy behaviors like eating
healthy, stopping smoking, and being aware of mental health.

Source: Office of Minority Health.

in Canada in 2011. With men not only dying earlier than women in Canada, but also
earlier than men in other areas of BC, the need to assess the reasons why was important
(Northern Health, 2011). The report used phone calls, interviews and focus groups with
men from the area to explore why men were not seeking out available preventive services
when compared to women. Men shared their challenges in accessing health care services
after hours, the influence of social and cultural expectations, the high-risk behaviors often
expected of men, such as drinking alcohol in excess, and the economic demands they
face to support their families (Northern Health, 2011). Although these issues are complex and multi-faceted, there were successful efforts that were highlighted in the report of
collaborations among community partners to meet the needs of men. Northern Health

also established DIGMA, or Doctor Initiated Group Medical Appointments, so that men could seek medical attention for specific health issues in groups with other men alongside them fostering a shared space to discuss medical concerns (2011).

Did you know?

In addition to the *Where are the men?* report, Northern Health BC (2013) created a video series to highlight additional examples of programs targeting men which included developing health pamphlets that compare maintaining health to maintaining a car with regular checkups, and programs in the winter for men to socialize and connect at the local gym while participating in group exercise classes. To watch part 1 of the series, visit www.youtube.com/watch?v=tzVrdXNXbs0. The remainder of the series is also available online.

Did you know?

When asked, "[n]early 81% of men remember the make & model of their first car, but barely half remember their last doctor visit."

(Man Cave Health, 2018, para. 2)

The report also included a recommendation for a comprehensive strategy to address men's health in northern BC by offering access to medical care through mobile clinics where men work and play, in addition to options at their home (Northern Health, 2011). Bringing mobile medical services to men allows them to participate in group screenings and educational programming (Northern Health, 2011). This approach necessitates the collaboration of multiple community partners, such as park and recreation centers and employers, thereby engaging the community level of the SEM in health promotion efforts. The authors of the report also recommend policy-level changes to support men, such as "policies regarding lengthened parental leave for new fathers, a living wage, income security, education and skills training for displaced workers, and family friendly workplaces [that] speak specifically to supporting men and their important role within society" (Northern Health, 2011, p. 58). This suggests that when communities, at both the local and national levels, use a comprehensive approach there can be improvements made to men's health.

Did you know?

Kayla Hense and photographer Thomas Brunot traveled across the United States to interview men on "the ways in which society, culture and personal experiences shape men's views of themselves" and their perspectives on masculinity (The Masculinity Project, n.d., para. 1). To learn more about their efforts, please visit https://themasculinityprojectus.com/.

How to use the book

Making the changes necessary to improve men's health around the world will take effort from everyone, including you, the reader. The resources and personal assessments that are included in each chapter can be helpful to anyone, regardless of their sex and gender. And if the information doesn't apply directly to you, perhaps you can use it to help the men close to you, or advocate for change on the local or national level. It benefits all when we address the needs of all. In the words of Dr. Jean Bonhomme (2016, p. 19), "men's health and women's health are not opposite ends of a seesaw. It's not either/or, it's both or neither."

Did you know?

International Men's Health Week takes place every June. For more information on men's health week events and for more information by country and/or regions, check out these links:

Australia: www.menshealthweek.org.au/
Europe: http://emhf.org/
New Zealand: www.menshealthweek.co.nz/
United States: www.menshealthnetwork.org

References

AHRQ. (2012). *Healthy men*. Retrieved from https://archive.ahrq.gov/patients-consumers/patient-involvement/healthy-men/index.html

Baker, P., Dworkin, S. L., Tong, S., Banks, I., Shand, T., & Yamey, G. (2014). The men's health gap: men must be included in the global health equity agenda. *Bulletin of the World Health Organization, 92*, 618–620.

Banks, I. (2001). No man's land: men, illness, and the NHS. *BMJ, 323*(7320), 1058–1060.

Bonhomme, J. (2016, January 8). *Defining and overcoming barriers: building bridges to men's health* [PowerPoint slides]. Retrieved from www.menshealthnetwork.org/dialogue/wp-content/uploads/2016/01/White-House-Dialogue-presentations.pdf

Centers for Disease Control and Prevention. (2015). *Suicide: facts at a glance, 2015*. Retrieved from www.cdc.gov/violenceprevention/pdf/suicide-datasheet-a.PDF

The Editors of Men's Health. (2015). *The most important thing you can do for your health today. A federal Office of Men's Health is needed to address the health risks of men—and you can help make it happen*. Retrieved from www.menshealth.com/health/a19548128/office-of-mens-health/

Fadich, A., Llamas, R. P., Giorgianni, S., Stephenson, C., & Nwaiwu, C. (2018). 2016 Survey of state-level health resources for men and boys: identification of an inadvertent and remediable service and health disparity. *American Journal of Men's Health, 12*(4), 1131–1137.

Gray, C. M., Hunt, K., Mutrie, N., Anderson, A. S., Leishman, J., Dalgarno, L., & Wyke, S. (2013). Football fans in training: the development and optimization of an intervention delivered through professional sports clubs to help men lose weight, become more active and adopt healthier eating habits. *BMC Public Health, 13*(1), 232.

Hasin, D. S., Stinson, F. S., Ogburn, E., & Grant, B. F. (2007). Prevalence, correlates, disability, and comorbidity of DSM-IV alcohol abuse and dependence in the United States: results from the National Epidemiologic Survey on Alcohol and Related Conditions. *Archives of General Psychiatry, 64*(7), 830–842.

Kilanowski, J. (2017). Breadth of the socio-ecological model. *Journal of Agromedicine, 22*(4), 295–297, DOI: 10.1080/1059924X.2017.1358971

Legato, M. J. (2019). *About us.* Retrieved from https://gendermed.org/about-us/

Man Cave Health. (2018). *About Man Cave Health.* Retrieved from https://mancavehealth.org/#about

The Masculinity Project. (n.d.). *The project.* Retrieved from https://themasculinityprojectus.com/read-me

Men's Health Forum. (n.d.). *Petition for a Men's Health Policy.* Retrieved from www.menshealthforum.org.uk/petition-mens-health-policy

Northern Health. (2011). *Where are the men? Chief Medical Health Officer's report on the health & well-being of men and boys in northern BC.* Retrieved from www.northernhealth.ca/sites/northern_health/files/about-us/reports/chief-mho-reports/documents/where-are-the-men.pdf

Northern Health BC. (2013, June 19). *Where are the men? Part 1 men's health documentary* [Video]. YouTube. www.youtube.com/watch?v=tzVrdXNXbs0

W. K. Kellogg Foundation. (2003). *Establishing an Office of Men's Health.* Retrieved from www.wkkf.org/~/media/D56269BC4D40474BA12C6EA2188F24EF.ashx

World Health Organization. (2019a). *Constitution.* Retrieved from www.who.int/about/who-we-are/constitution

World Health Organization. (2019b). *The Ottawa Charter for Health Promotion.* Retrieved from www.who.int/healthpromotion/conferences/previous/ottawa/en/

2 Masculinity and seeking help

Norman Eburne

Gender inequality is an irrefutable fact and in many aspects of life it makes it more diffi-cult for women to cope and thrive. In the case of health, however, it is likewise hard to be a man (Hawkes & Buse, 2013). Men can expect to live fewer years than women and are afflicted with a greater number of illnesses that diminish their quality of life (Bonhomme, Brott & Fadich, 2017). Throughout much of the developed world males do not fare as well as females in most measures of health, as well as length of life. According to the World Health Organization (WHO), by 2016, women were outliving men by an average of about six years. This ranged from 5.3 years in sub-Saharan Africa to 11.6 years in the Russian Federation (WHO, 2016). According to the Centers for Disease Control and Prevention (2019) women live about five years longer than men in the United States (81.1 to 76.1). In the United Kingdom, 20% of men die prior to their 65th birthday, but after that their death rate is roughly equal to that of women (Rochelle, Yeung, Bond & Li, 2015).

Part of the reason why men are less healthy and live for a shorter period of time is thought to be that men are less diligent in seeking or utilizing health care, and that premise has merit. Compared to women, men are about 25% less likely to have seen a health care provider over the last year, 50% less likely over a two-year period and three times less likely over a five-year period (Smith, Braunack-Mayer & Wittert, 2006). This avoidance of seeking care may be a major factor in men's health problems.

In his own words

Dave, former college heavyweight wrestler and football defensive lineman
"You have really done it this time" were the thoughts running through my head as I laid in the hospital bed awaiting my toe amputation. How does a college educated man with a health degree nonetheless, put himself in this spot? The ordeal started about six weeks earlier when I started noticing the swelling and redness around the toe. I dealt with it as I had with any previous infection in my body. As a rough and tough country boy who rarely went to the doctor, this was just a little bump in the road I thought. Not to mention I had a big hunting and fishing trip I was looking forward to. The toe didn't get any worse so I didn't really give it much thought as I prepared for my journey across the country to hunt and fish in Louisiana. While on the trip the toe swelled up. When I arrived back in Oregon I knew I had to get to the doctor. It was determined that the infection had gotten into the bone and the best course of action was to remove it. Being the second toe, it would not impact my active lifestyle too much and fortunately it hasn't. The question is why

didn't I go to the doctor right away, being that I have good insurance and am in a good spot financially? I would guess it is a combination of how I was raised, ego-driven and stubbornness. I was raised that you didn't go to the doctor unless it is life threatening. I am a college educated man with a degree in health and spent a ton of time in sports medicine type classes, so probably thought I knew more than I really did. The third factor was I am probably just stubborn. I have always prided myself on being tougher than most people. The combination of these factors led me to not getting checked out until it was too late to save the toe.

Compared to women, men are much less focused on prevention or early diagnosis and treatment of health problems. Men avoid going to the doctor, skip recommended screenings and practice riskier behavior than do women. This likely contributes to the premature death and higher illness rates. For every ten premature deaths by women pre age 50, 16 men will die prematurely from such things as cardiovascular disease, cancer, unintentional injuries and suicide (Addis & Mahalik, 2003). Obtaining help for health concerns involves recognizing that there may be a problem, then seeking and utilizing the assistance of an appropriate health care provider. Generally, men do this less frequently than women and are more likely to terminate therapy early (Parent, Hammer, Bradstreet, Schwartz & Jobe, 2018). This neglect of health care extends to dental health. Furuta et al. (2011) report that women are almost twice as likely as men to have had a dental exam in the past year. It is believed that this is responsible for women having less dental plaque, calculus and bleeding upon dental probing.

Learn more

Man Up, an Australian program that includes a website, blog and television series, released a one-minute campaign ad titled "Why do we tell boys to stop crying?" highlighting the social and cultural expectations placed upon men and boys when experiencing emotional pain. To learn more, visit http://manup.org.au/tv-series/campaign-ad/.

Factors impacting men seeking health care

Tudiver and Talbot (1999) sought the opinion of family physicians, as to why men tend to underuse primary health care services even though they become sick more often and die earlier. Responding physicians described three key themes involved in avoiding or under-utilizing care. The first involved *support*. Men tend to get most of their support regarding health concerns from female partners, rather than male friends (Tudiver & Talbot, 1999). A study conducted by the Cleveland Clinic (2018) revealed that 83% of women surveyed said that they attempted to encourage male partners to have a health checkup each year. However, 30% of male respondents to the survey agreed with the statement "I don't need annual health checks with a doctor, I'm healthy" (Cleveland Clinic, 2018).

Furthermore, Ek (2013) revealed that Finnish men were not inclined to seek or discuss health-related information. The difference between Finnish men and women differed at statistically significant levels when it came to discussing health matters. Men were not as interested in world-wide health issues or how food, shelter and other goods affected their health, and they viewed knowledge about health as a woman's role in the family and that women should be gatekeepers and custodians of the family's health (Ek, 2013).

The second theme involved viewing *help seeking* as something that might make them appear vulnerable. Fear that something may be wrong or denial of symptoms were reported as factors inhibiting help seeking (Tudiver & Talbot, 1999). Men tend to look for help for specific problems rather than for general concerns or routine inspections (Tudiver & Talbot, 1999). The third theme involved personal *barriers* that relate to perceived traditional male roles and attributes. These include a sense of immunity to problems, feelings of immortality, difficulty relinquishing control and a belief that seeking help was unacceptable (Tudiver & Talbot, 1999).

Research by Taber, Leyva and Persoskie (2015) identified other barriers, including unfavorable past experiences with health care that involved the physician or some aspect of the health care organization. Traditional barriers such as cost, lack of insurance or time constraints were given by 58.4% of those surveyed (Taber et al., 2015). A Brazilian study by Patrão et al. (2017) identified similar barriers for men. Specifically, women report and respond to illness more readily while men tended to refuse to respond as readily to illness and men regarded responding to illness as a denial of virility and believed it was more in keeping with manhood to endure pain in silence (Patrão et al., 2017).

Personal assessment

The American Heart Association has identified ten reasons why men do not seek out health care (2018). These include:

1. not having a doctor
2. not having insurance
3. not believing that there is a need to see a doctor
4. not having available time
5. not wanting to pay for health care services
6. not understanding the role of a doctor
7. not being ready to hear a diagnosis
8. not wanting a physical exam
9. not seeing a value in seeing a doctor
10. not wanting to follow my partner's advice to get a checkup

How many of these can you relate to?

Learn more

While not specific to the issue of healthcare, *The Masculine Self*, 6th Edition, written by Andrew P. Smiler and Christopher Kilmartin does explore the role of masculinities in the lives of boys and men.

Masculinity and health care

Men are often faulted for downplaying the degree of pain or disability associated with an illness or health problem. The social construction of maleness plays a role in how men interpret or react to departures from optimal health (Moore & Gillette, 2013). Some observers have gone so far as to suggest that masculine culture and values are hazardous to their health. The development of maleness is often associated with adherence to patriarchal, masculine attributes including dominance, self-reliance, superiority and independence. These are all attributes that would impede the desire to seek medical care. Men are accused of being poor consumers of health services and thus victims of their own attitudes and choices. But is a "piling on" of the men behaving badly charge any more than victim blaming? It might be more helpful to examine the intersection of typical male personality patterns and the health care system if the ultimate goal is to encourage men to recognize the need for help and to follow up by seeking and utilizing it.

Cleary (2005) describes four male personality types that take a less than positive view of masculinity. These include career type masculinity, enterprising masculinity, family-oriented/breadwinner masculinity, and pure scientific masculinity. Review each type in Table 2.1 and consider how each would influence involvement with health care.

Just how men get to be the way they are has much to do with how they are mentored into manhood. How is this done? Who is involved? What are the outcomes? There are many examples of the initiation process for young men found in various cultures around the world. Some of these involve a symbolic rebirth into a male subculture. Very often they involve acts of bravery such as engaging in battle, hunting or enduring pain. Joining an athletic team and falling under the influence of a male figure coach, or accompanying his father or a band of men to kill his first deer are common examples in some countries. But most involve some form of leaving their mother's nurturing and influence in order to begin associating with and adopting the characteristics and behavior patterns of men.

Modern western society has symbolic vestiges of manhood initiation ceremonies. Entering the military and completing basic training, or hazing as part of the initiation rituals of a college fraternity can serve a similar purpose. Most of these rituals take the young male and put him under the leadership of an older strong male figure. Signs of weakness, such as responding to pain or discomfort are not valued during this process. From a study of members of the Canadian military, Roberge (2007) noted that masculinity was a highly prized attribute and that a successful military man was expected to be competitive, invulnerable, determined and brave. He was expected to not cry, not to be hurt or reveal pain,

Table 2.1 Male personality types and descriptions

Masculinity type	Description
Career type masculinity	Places maximum interest on career and minimum interest on family relationships
Enterprising masculinity	Attempts to couple a high degree of focus on both career and a positive relationship with the family
Family-oriented/ breadwinner masculinity	Low concern or emphasis on career and very high emphasis on family relationships
Pure scientific masculinity	Minimal focus on both career and family

Source: Male personality types as described by Cleary (2005), developed by chapter author.

not to be listed as sick and not to ask for leave to travel home (Roberge, 2007). In his book *Sea Stories: My life in special operations*, Admiral William H. McRaven (2019) states that the number one attribute that U.S. Navy Seals garner in training is that no matter what, they do not quit. A Russian description of a *real man* (Zinn, 1982) is someone who is expected to pursue victory, take risks, struggle, lead and achieve success. In addition to the *real man*, there exists *natural masculinity* which exhibits different attributes that do not allow for a crisis or failure of manhood.

A term frequently used to describe men in a negative light is macho or machismo. One use of the term is to describe proud, arrogant, self-serving, female-dominating behavior. The "macho man" brings to mind the picture of a strutting rooster attempting to bolster a flagging ego. However, a less derogatory application of the term uses it to describe a man who gets out of bed at 4:30 a.m. to travel to a job in the rain or hot sun that offers poor financial reward and less prestige. An interesting example of machismo is the man who swallows his pride, ignores belittling glances or comments and persists in a difficult job in order to provide for his family. It is up to each individual to determine which def-inition is acceptable. But before deciding on a definition, or glibly using the term as an insult, it's important to take the opportunity to observe male workers, often of immigrant or minority status and evaluate the level of dignity in some of their stoic, self-sacrificing behavior.

There have been many attempts to study, describe and explain masculinity. The term hegemonic masculinity describes efforts by men to compete vigorously and attempt to gain and maintain a dominance over females, as well as other males (Connell & Messerschmidt, 2005). Just as the term macho often camouflages the complexity of male identity, many observers recognized that hegemonic masculinity was too broad a label to be fairly applied to a cross-section of complex male behavior. There are many types of masculinity that influence a variety of activities, including seeking and utilizing health care. As you read a very brief description of some of the types of masculinity, ask yourself which ones have some bearing on male health-related behavior.

- *Hegemonic masculinity* is based on traditional male roles and privileges that tend to legitimize the patriarchy (George, 2006). It involves great emphasis on physical strength, dominating others, suppressing emotions and tolerating pain. It rejects help as a way to assert masculinity. Behaving like a man would mean to downplay self-care and health needs in order to portray males as being stronger than females.
- *Toxic masculinity* describes a male who exhibits the need to aggressively compete with and dominate others. This overemphasis on traditional male roles can inhibit the expression of emotions that might otherwise be normal in boys and men. Bullying and domestic violence are examples of toxic masculinity. Connell & Messerschmidt (2005) believe that this is a behavioral pattern that extends out from hegemonic masculinity.
- *Precarious masculinity* suggests that dominating manhood is not innate but can be achieved. This often involves a ritual initiation. Boys have undergone, often painful, rituals in order to be considered real men. Manhood may also be lost when a man is considered by others to "not be manly enough" (Vandello, Bosson, Cohen, Burnaford & Weaver, 2008). Being overly concerned about seeking help for injuries or other health problems may be a sufficient social transgression to cause loss of perceived manhood. In such cases, men would likely take some action to demonstrate their ability to work through or "tough out" a problem without seeking help.

These brief descriptions of various modes of male-oriented behavior could be expanded to an extremely complex and unwieldy degree. A different perspective is the *inclusive masculinity theory*, which views masculinity as being influenced by social changes that have undermined traditional hegemonic masculinity and its anti-woman and homo-phobic tenets (Vandello et al., 2008). In the past, these tenets have caused men to avoid behavior that might reflect a more emotional, gentle side of themselves in order to avoid being perceived as soft or gay. As society evolves and progresses, new spaces are opening where men can be accepted and thrive without the need to behave in hypermasculine ways. When this occurs, men will be able to engage in a variety of behaviors previously considered feminine without fear of being perceived as weak or gay. Such advances, hope-fully, will include acceptance of appropriate use of preventive and therapeutic health care.

Did you know?

The Men's Health Network (n.d.) offers a checklist of recommended screenings for men, detailing the recommended age range and frequency for the tests. To learn more, visit www.menshealthnetwork.org/library/getitcheckedpostermen.pdf.

Men, relationships and health care

In his work, *Manhood in the Making*, David Gilmore (1990) describes the three P's of manhood. These are *Protect*, *Procreate* and *Provide*. Gilmore argues that most of the world's cultures or societies have ascribed these or very similar roles to those who would assume traditional roles of manhood. One of the P's, to *Procreate*, doesn't have much to do with this chapter other than that men who procreate large families are more likely to be in a position to deny themselves the expense and/or time associated with professional health care due to the need to spread resources further. The other P's, *Provide* and *Protect*, may be more related to the issue at hand. Traditionally the protector required physical skill, courage and stoicism to be effective. In modern times, the protector would be more likely to sacrifice himself or his own needs to care for those he is protecting. This might entail purchasing an SUV rather than a sports sedan for family transportation, or forgoing football season tickets in order to fund a family vacation. The provider has always been called upon to be self-reliant and competent in seeking materials for food and shelter plus demonstrating a willingness to share a larger portion of the spoils with others. With the coming of the industrial age, the provider left home for long hours each day to partici-pate in such efforts as mining or manufacturing just as sailors, hunters or fishermen had done in earlier times. In all cases, the successful provider would present major portions of his reward to the family. This notion of a man's role can easily be extrapolated to con-temporary men delaying or avoiding seeking help in exchange for the opportunity to do more for the family.

Kipnis (as cited in Pascoe, 2003) reports a client who, when going through his finances, discovered that during the previous year, when his earnings were well in excess of $100,000, he had spent less than $1,200 on himself. During that same year, his wife had exceeded $10,000 in psychological therapy and his children had spent more on optional health issues. This disparity in financial expenditures is an example of some men's reluc-tance to expend money on health care for themselves.

The Pew Research Center (Parker & Stepler, 2017) reports that in spite of gender equity advances, in more than 65% of married or cohabiting couples in the United States, the male partner earns the greater portion of the family income. Americans continue to regard the man as the key financial provider even as women's contributions grow. Seventy-one percent of people surveyed said it is important for a man to be able to support the family financially and to be a good provider (Parker & Stepler, 2017). This cultural pressure causes men to place a greater emphasis on their role as provider. African American and Hispanic men are more likely than Caucasians to place a high level of importance on being able to financially support a family. Even if a worker's health care is covered by insurance, there are still copayments and deductible costs associated with health care. Additionally, paid leave usually does not cover time taken off work to visit a physician. The loss of a day's pay can be a deterrent to seeking care.

Men and how they experience pain

The reason that men seek health care less frequently than women may also have a physical basis. Evidence exists to suggest that men do not feel or respond to pain as well as women do (Rosseland & Stubhaug, 2004). Differences in subjective responses to pain between men and women have been consistently reported (Keogh & Herdenfeldt, 2002). The bulk of the research into a biological basis of pain reveals that men experience less pain, have less pain-related distress and less response to experimentally induced pain. More to the point, the heightened pain threshold and tolerance levels in men means that they likely do not interpret the discomfort associated with an injury or impending illness as well as women. When men respond to an injury or illness by saying "It's nothing" or "I'm O.K." they may be being honest. This could be a major factor in men not reporting a problem or seeking help in remedying it.

Did you know?

Mantherapy.org (2019) features a *Head Inspection* self-assessment and offers users multiple resources on a wide variety of men's health issues, such as depression, anger and grief. To learn more, visit Mantherapy.org.

Moving forward

In earlier societies the male role was to be protector and provider. Why this developed isn't clear, but it may have been due to the larger size and strength of men coupled with a tendency to take greater risks. The aggression-promoting effect of testosterone may have also played a role. For whatever reason, perhaps none of the above, men have assumed and accepted the fixer, provider, leader role in most societies or cultures. This became, rather than a biology-based role, a sociocultural-influenced, assumed and even expected role for the male. Whatever the reason, this dynamic became the norm in the majority of human societies. Late 20th- and early 21st-century reasoning and enlightenment has modified gender roles in the direction of equitable contribution. However there remain vestiges of earlier roles and responsibilities for men. But for many, concepts of bravery, self-denial and other behaviors described earlier in the chapter still linger and lie buried in the male mode of thinking. This could be a prime mover in men's avoidance or lesser use of the health care system.

While the major global health institutions are mostly aware of the problems associated with men and incomplete or ineffective health care, they still seem to assume that the largest need for improvement in health care delivery applies to women (McKinlay, Kljakovic & McBain, 2009). With the exceptions of Australia, Brazil and Ireland, national government health programs tend to minimize the need to reduce the illness burden carried by men, if not ignore it completely. Efforts to lighten the global burden of disease and improve public health should focus on the needs of all genders.

From a global perspective, Manandhar, Hawkes, Buse, Nosrati and Magar (2018) have identified several ways that countries can address the gender inequities in health care. One of these recommendations is to understand the social roles that accompany gender within a specific society, and how that impacts health care access and usage.

In the United States, the Affordable Care Act (ACA; sometimes known as ObamaCare) was designed and implemented in an effort to assure that all people had access to quality health care with no financial barriers. Soon after implementation of the ACA, several million previously uninsured or underinsured residents of the country had affordable and effective health insurance. The Act was a significant advance as a starting point toward even better results, but like many large programs initiated there were some deficiencies. Some of the shortcomings involved administrative and organizational structure that furthered obstacles to men accessing health care (obamacarefacts.com, 2018). The ACA prohibits discrimination on the basis of race, color, national origin, sex, age or disability. But in reality, girls and women are covered for a variety of services not available to boys or men. In the design of the ACA, women younger than 24 years of age as well as other high-risk women were to receive free screening for chlamydia and all sexually active women could avail themselves of free gonorrhea screening. While these tests are equally effective for both genders, men were not guaranteed such screenings as a benefit. Breast cancer screening was provided without a required copayment or coinsurance while screening for prostate cancer (a leading male cancer) did not come with the same financial incentive. The ACA requires plans to pay for counselling and contraception for women. Covered contraceptive methods include implanted devices, oral contraception, barrier methods and emergency contraception (morning after pill) plus voluntary sterilization procedures. With regard to male contraception, the ACA did not require insurers to pay for vasectomies, or even condoms. The Act offers paid Well Women visits but no similar programs for men. The ACA has a specific chapter devoted to women's health but nothing similar regarding men's health (Bedsider, 2018). The ACA lists 134 references specific to women's health and two references directed toward men's health. While these inconsistencies between male- and female-oriented aspects of the United States' first attempt at a national health insurance program may not be a barrier to men accessing or using care, they certainly are far from a form of encouragement. Even domestic violence care is not covered equitably in the ACA. Men are not covered for violence screening, while women are. The fact that the ACA has so many female-oriented benefits is a very good thing and should be supported to the fullest. The issue here is that men are not afforded the same level of preventive care and that male-oriented programs are not as well promoted. To some, the message may be that men's health in the United States is less important and this chapter is attempting to remedy that.

References

Addis, M. E., & Mahalik, J. R. (2003). Men, masculinity, and the contexts of help seeking. *American Psychologist, 58*(1), 5.

American Heart Association. (2018). *The top 10 reasons men put off doctor visits.* Retrieved from www.heart.org/HEARTORG/Conditions/Heart-Disease-PUT-OFF-DOCTORVISITS_UCM_433365_Article.jsp#.Xe2bRpNKgkh

Bedsider. (2018, November 1). *Men's health and the Affordable Care Act: What's covered?* Retrieved from www.bedsider.org/features/862-men-s-health-and-the-affordable-care-act-what-s-covered

Bonhomme, L., Brott, A., & Fadich, A. (2017, December 20). *Why men don't care about the health care debate.* Retrieved from www.statnews.com/2017/12/20/ men-health-care-debate/

Centers for Disease Control and Prevention. (2019). *Life expectancy at selected ages by sex: United States, 2016 and 2017 [Fact Sheet].* Retrieved from www.cdc.gov/nchs/data/factsheets/factsheet_NVSS.pdf

Cleary, A. (2005). Death rather than disclosure: struggling to be a real man. *Irish Journal of Sociology, 14*(2), 155–176.

Cleveland Clinic. (2018, Sept. 5). *Cleveland Clinic Survey: Spouses/significant others play an influential role in getting men to take their health seriously.* [Press Release]. Retrieved from https://newsroom.clevelandclinic.org/2018/09/05/cleveland-clinic-survey-spouses-significant-others-play-an-influential-role-in-getting-men-to-take-their-health-seriously/

Connell, R. W., & Messerschmidt, J. W. (2005). Hegemonic masculinity: rethinking the concept. *Gender & Society, 19*(6), 829–859.

Ek, S. (2013). Gender differences in health information behaviour: a Finnish population-based survey. *Health Promotion International, 30*(3), 736–745.

Furuta, M., Ekuni, D., Irie, K., Azuma, T., Tomofuji, T., Ogura, T., & Morita, M. (2011). Sex differences in gingivitis relate to interaction of oral health behaviors in young people. *Journal of Periodontology, 82*(4), 558–565.

George, A. (2006). Reinventing honorable masculinity: discourses from a working-class Indian community. *Men and Masculinities, 9*(1), 35–52.

Gilmore, D. D. (1990). *Manhood in the Making: Cultural concepts of masculinity.* Yale University Press.

Hawkes, S., & Buse, K. (2013). Gender and global health: evidence, policy, and inconvenient truths. *The Lancet, 381*(9879), 1783–1787.

Keogh, E., & Herdenfeldt, M. (2002). Gender, coping and the perception of pain. *Pain, 97*(3), 195–201.

Manandhar, M., Hawkes, S., Buse, K., Nosrati, E., & Magar, V. (2018). Gender, health and the 2030 agenda for sustainable development. *Bulletin of the World Health Organization, 96*(9), 644.

Mantherapy.org (2019). *Welcome to man therapy.* Retrieved from www.mantherapy.org/

McKinlay, E., Kljakovic, M., & McBain, L. (2009). New Zealand men's health care: are we meeting the needs of men in general practice? *Journal of Primary Health Care, 1*(4), 302–310.

McRaven, W. H. (2019). *Sea Stories: My life in special operations.* Grand Central Publishing.

Men's Health Network. (n.d.). *Men: get it checked.* Retrieved from www.menshealthnetwork.org/library/getitcheckedpostermen.pdf

Moore, R., & Gillette, D. (2013). *King, Warrior, Magician, Lover: Rediscovering the archetypes of the mature masculine.* HarperCollins Publishers.

obamacarefacts.com. (2018, October 1). *ObamaCare and women: ObamaCare women's health services. ObamaCare fact.* Retrieved from https://obamacarefacts.com/obamacare-womens-health-services/

Parent, M. C., Hammer, J. H., Bradstreet, T. C., Schwartz, E. N., & Jobe, T. (2018). Men's mental health help-seeking behaviors: an intersectional analysis. *American Journal of Men's Health, 12*(1), 64–73.

Parker, K., & Stepler, R. (2017, Sept. 20). Americans see men as the financial providers, even as women's contributions grow. *Pew Research Center.*

Pascoe, C. J. (2003). Multiple masculinities? Teenage boys talk about jocks and gender. *American Behavioral Scientist, 46*(10), 1423–1438.

Patrão, A. L., da Conceição Almeida, M., Matos, S. M. A., Chor, D., & Aquino, E. M. (2017). Gender and psychosocial factors associated with healthy lifestyle in the Brazilian Longitudinal Study of Adult Health (ELSA-Brasil) cohort: a cross-sectional study. *BMJ Open, 7*(8), e015705.

Roberge, J. (2007). *Les stratégies de coping utilisées par les militaires ou ex-militaires masculins atteints d'un stress post-traumatique suite au retour d'une mission de paix.* École de service social, Faculté des sciences sociales, Université Laval, Quebec City, Quebec.

Rochelle, T. L., Yeung, D. K., Bond, M. H., & Li, L. M. W. (2015). Predictors of the gender gap in life expectancy across 54 nations. *Psychology, Health & Medicine, 20*(2), 129–138.

Rosseland, L. A., & Stubhaug, A. (2004). Gender is a confounding factor in pain trials: women report more pain than men after arthroscopic surgery. *Pain, 112*(3), 248–253.

Smiler, A., & Kilmartin, C. (2018). *The Masculine Self*, 6th ed. Sloan Publishing.

Smith, J., Braunack-Mayer, A., & Wittert, G. (2006). What do we know about men's help-seeking and health service use? *Medical Journal of Australia, 184*(2), 81–83.

Taber, J. M., Leyva, B., & Persoskie, A. (2015). Why do people avoid medical care? A qualitative study using national data. *Journal of General Internal Medicine, 30*(3), 290–297.

Tudiver, F., & Talbot, Y. (1999). Why don't men seek help? Family physicians' perspectives on help-seeking behavior in men. *Journal of Family Practice, 48*, 47–52.

Vandello, J. A., Bosson, J. K., Cohen, D., Burnaford, R. M., & Weaver, J. R. (2008). Precarious manhood. *Journal of Personality and Social Psychology, 95*(6), 1325.

World Health Organization. (2016). *World Health Statistics 2016: monitoring health for the SDGs.* Retrieved from www.who.int/gho/publications/world_health_statistics/2016/en/

Zinn, M. B. (1982). Chicano men and masculinity. *The Journal of Ethnic Studies, 10*(2), 29.

3 Body image

James E. Leone

Body image dissatisfaction can have profound effects on people, particularly the under-studied population of males. This chapter will explore the intersectionality of male gender and body image.

In his own words

Drew was raised in a middle class midwestern family. He had an older brother and a younger sister and both parents were present in his life. Drew's father was a football coach and his older brother Ethan was a football player and powerlifter. Drew was never really drawn to sports or competition-based sports more specifically. Being relatively smaller through adolescence (he was 5 feet 5 inches and 125 lb), Drew often wished to be bigger and more on par with his male peers. Although never bullied, he was always sensitive to comments regarding being "small" or "weaker looking." In fact, Drew's dad often would jokingly remark on his size calling him "slim" and "goose neck." When Drew graduated he began to explore exercise and weight training; and in addition to the normal course of growth and development, he reached a height of 6 feet and weighed approximately 165 lb. Drew wanted more, he wanted to look like the guys on fitness magazines! Drew tried all sorts of supplements, diets, work out plans, and spent a significant portion of his earnings on these endeavors. He even hired a personal trainer to the tune of $600 per month! He was never really happy with his physical progress even though others often would remark on how built he was ... he was convinced he needed more. Drew's obsession with exercise and his looks greatly impacted his job and relationships as he would sacrifice them in favor of looking better.

Overview

Body image has been formally defined as "the internal, subjective representations of physical appearance and bodily experience" (Philips, 1998, p. 199) and is a complex, multidimensional construct of the human experience. How one *sees* himself is a function of when, how, and with whom he interacts in society as well as appraisals that are internalized by the individual from these experiences (Davis & Cowles, 1991).

Consistent trends prevail concerning body image dissatisfaction in the United States and abroad (Hrabosky et al., 2009). Annually, billions of consumer dollars are spent with hopes of addressing body image concerns, such as overweight, fatness, muscularity, and cosmetic beauty among others (Leit, Gray, & Pope, 2002; Sarwer et al., 2005; Sarwer & Polonsky, 2016). Researchers note that "supplement industries and the media have made billions by capitalizing on our insecurities with our bodies" (Pope, Phillips, & Olivardia, 2000, p. 242). Pope, Khalsa, and Bhasin (2017) have studied various global cultural shifts in male body image and the connection to performance-enhancing substances, body image drugs, and androgenic-anabolic steroids. Overall, they note a steadily growing and heightened dissatisfaction with body image ranging from Europe and North America to Australia, South Africa, and even Samoa (Pope, Gruber, et al., 2000).

Development of body image is dependent on several social influences, but also unique innate individual qualities. The relationship with a negative body image often fuels negative behaviors, such as eating disorders, disordered eating patterns, low self-esteem, risky sexual practices, and crash dieting, among others (Dakanalis et al., 2013). Understanding what factors promote or inhibit the development of a healthy body image is imperative at a young age via parental modeling and is particularly critical considering the increasing social value of idealism of the physique, males notwithstanding.

Perhaps the most commonplace examples as to why people, particularly adolescents, seem to be more focused than ever on how they look, is the result of media influences (Fardouly & Vartarnian, 2016). Media is an omnipresent and omnipotent factor in daily life. For many men, media convinces them that they are simply not good enough and that they can always improve (Sarwer & Polonsky, 2016). Many industries, such as supplement companies, thrive off making people feel insecure with their bodies (Pope, Phillips, et al., 2000). Rather than celebrating endless human variety, unscrupulous companies aim at capitalizing on people's insecurities in the name of profit. Certainly, much attention pertaining to body image has been skewed toward women; however, increasingly, attention also has been dedicated to men. The next section will explore how body image in males has evolved in the context of social norms and the resulting physical and psycho-emotional consequences.

Research with men

Concern for body image was never absent in males, but rather, not brought to the surface of public consciousness and dialogue. Male body image concerns have only surfaced in the past couple of decades (Mangweth et al., 2004; Pope, Phillips, et al., 2000). Recent trends of male preoccupation with physical appearance and the impact on body image and cognitive affect has led to new insights concerning the depth of the issue, but also strategies to mitigate negative effects (Dakanalis et al., 2013). For example, college campuses and clinical settings are more apt to encourage mental health well-being, positive body image, and self-care regardless of gender (Halliwell, 2015).

Variations among cultures and global perspectives have been studied in men as well, with trends indicating body image dissatisfaction occurs in countries with a similar socioeconomic status as the United States (e.g., United Kingdom, Israel, Austria, Australia, Samoa) (Franko et al., 2015; Lipinski & Pope, 2002; Pope, Gruber, et al., 2000). Similar to television consumption detailed by Tiggeman (2005) and also Baghurst, Hollander, Nardella, and Haff (2006) assert that modeling through toy action figures, such as G.I. Joe and Marvel™ superheroes, may contribute to body dissatisfaction or distortion in boys and men. In this research, action figures were found to have become hypermuscular over time (1960s to the 2000s) far exceeding the muscularity of even the largest bodybuilders.

A similar trend also was noted in *Playgirl* male centerfold models from the 1970s through the 1990s as well as other women's magazines (Pope, Olivardia, Borowiecki, & Cohane, 2001). These factors may contribute to the development of spectrum and somatoform disorders, such as body dysmorphia or muscle dysmorphia, to be discussed in following sections. These trends contribute to a contemporary paradox of males wanting to be heavier, but perceiving themselves as lighter (Pope, Phillips, et al., 2000).

Men, like women, often want to change their weight, but often are more preoccupied with body shape and muscularity (Grogan, 2016). Appearance often is equated to success and with terms such as, metrosexual, today's man often finds a need to react to these pressures. Reactions vary but may include: obsessive exercise, dieting, use of body image drugs (Dakanalis et al., 2013; Kanayama, Pope, & Hudson, 2001), and even cosmetic surgery (Westmoreland-Corson & Anderson, 2004).

Research with boys and adolescent males

Body image is the most important component of an adolescent's global self-esteem (Graber, Peterson, & Brooks-Gunn, 1996). Similarly, globally, concern for body image appears to be a strong factor in developed societies (Pope, Gruber, et al., 2000), whereas underdeveloped and developing nations report less concern (Franko et al., 2015). This point tends to reflect Abraham Maslow's hierarchy of needs, such as basic needs must be met before other secular concerns become an issue. Masculine beauty is less easily defined, although trends toward a more muscular physique are preferred by males according to existing and recent evidence (Leone et al., 2011, 2015; Pope, Phillips, et al., 2000).

As boys and girls mature (roughly to age 11), both typically show comparable levels of overall body esteem through childhood (Field et al., 1999). Several studies indicate trends of dissatisfaction with body shape and weight in elementary school children and adolescent boys (Field et al., 1999; Leone et al., 2011; Ricciardelli & McCabe, 2001). Forty percent of elementary school girls and 25% of boys expressed discontent when measured with a modified body image satisfaction instrument (Field et al., 1999). Children as young as six years of age have been found to express concern with their bodies (Ricciardelli & McCabe, 2001). Internalization of negative affect at a young age appears to be a strong predictor of body image disturbance in adolescence and into adulthood.

Underweight boys are most likely to be dissatisfied with their body image and many with normal weight wish to weigh more (Dion et al., 2016; Leone et al., 2011). Boys often desire larger upper arms, chest, and shoulders, with approximately one-third reporting being dissatisfied with their body shape (Dion et al., 2016). Exercise is more likely to be chosen than dieting and purging by boys as methods of weight control (Grogan, 2016). Dieting among boys is more likely to be associated with increased body weight and some sports, such as wrestling (Grogan, 2016; Kanayama et al., 2001).

Body satisfaction in boys decreases from elementary school years through adolescence (Cohane & Pope, 2001; Grogan, 2016). Often, this trend reverses as boys progress through puberty due to gains in muscle mass. Weight gain associated with lean mass is perceived as positive for adolescent males (Cohane & Pope, 2001). Younger males often report wanting to be bigger with respect to muscle mass. For example, Gruber and Pope (1999) presented a computer-based body image program to younger males with results showing that males preferred a heavier physique when compared to what they believe to be ideal. When males were asked to select from a group of silhouettes, they tended to select a heavier-than-average silhouette. This trend appears consistent likely because boys equate *heavier* with more *muscular* in the absence of a silhouette that clearly represents *muscular*. When compared to female perspectives of ideal male physiques, results consistently demonstrated a much higher body weight ideal from the male perspective (Gruber & Pope, 1999).

Because adolescence is a period of emotional, social, psychological, and physical change, feelings of discontent may result in negative health behaviors, ranging from dieting and cosmetic surgeries to other compensatory behaviors (Kanayama et al., 2001; Sarwer & Polonsky, 2016). Males typically gain upwards of 75 to 100 pounds with lean muscle mass as the majority, but those who do not, or do not meet sociocultural standards, may become dissatisfied (Grogan, 2016; Leone et al., 2011; Pope, Phillips, et al., 2000). This model sets up a paradigm for potential male body image dissatisfaction because of a lack of adequate gain and/or weight distribution. Puberty does not consistently correlate to body image dissatisfaction; however, it does accentuate previous existing vulnerabilities and problems, such as low self-esteem and feelings of shame. Timing may play a major role, with early development as a positive factor for males and late development (commonly referred to as a late bloomer) as a negative factor for males (Leone et al., 2015).

Male body image and self-esteem

In its basic sense, self-esteem is a person's thoughts or beliefs about their value or worth. Formally, self-esteem is defined as a feeling of pride in oneself as it relates to global image as well as the congruence with a desired image of oneself. Self-esteem is inherently related to body image. Higher or lower levels of self-esteem have been suggested to directly impact a person's perception of their body image (Grogan, 2016). Dissatisfaction with body image has been linked to lower levels of self-esteem (Cash, 2004; Lubans et al., 2016). An etiological pathway that can lead to eating disturbances and, potentially, eating disorders, such as anorexia nervosa (AN) and bulimia nervosa (BN) is conceptualized in Figure 3.1.

The male body is often viewed in terms of its functionality. Loss of functionality or perceptions of diminished functionality may negatively impact self-esteem and subsequently body image, thus leading to negative behaviors (Grogan, 2016). Comments and criticism have both direct and indirect influences on a person's self-esteem, perceived self-efficacy, and ultimately body image. Direct insults or negative criticism often have a dramatic impact; however, indirect comments, criticism, and social influences often evolve over time, which may lead to an overall drastic change in a person's self-esteem (Evans, Roy, Geiger, Werner, & Burnett, 2008). For example, a friend may openly criticize

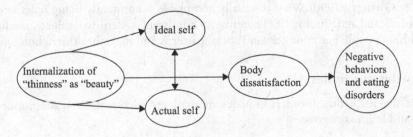

Figure 3.1 Etiologic pathway to eating disturbances.
Source: Adapted from Striegel-Moore & Franko (2004).

another, leading the person to question their self-image; this would be an instance of direct negative criticism. Indirect negative criticism accumulates over time; for example, comments by a parent or close relative about a person's body weight, often builds over time leading to a negative body image.

Relationship among the media, advertising, and body image

Social marketing and targeted marketing strategies play a strong role in how people perceive their body image. Constant exposure to these social factors plays a key reinforcing role for each message or advertisement, whether positive or negative in content (Fardouly & Vartarnian, 2016; Grogan, 2016). Time of exposure and media consumption patterns as well as type of content were studied by Holland and Tiggemann (2016). Results suggested that although time of exposure reinforces the marketing message, the content of the material played a greater role in the development of negative feelings toward one's body. Males who are bombarded with idealistic and unrealistic images of a hypermasculine ideal likely will pursue maladaptive behaviors (e.g. dieting, supplements, body image drugs, etc.).

The use of uncommonly fit models is another trend in current media, which may impact a person's body image (Holland & Tiggemann, 2016; Tiggemann, 2005). Social comparison theory states that humans are likely to compare based on current status and idealistic thoughts, and this is particularly true of boys and men. When a discrepancy is noted based on the comparison, discord arises that often motivates a person to take action. Negative health actions (behaviors) may include extreme dieting practices, use of excessive dietary supplements, unhealthy exercise patterns, or even full-blown eating disorders (Dakanalis et al., 2013; Grogan, 2016; Holland & Tiggemann, 2016; Kanayama et al., 2001; Tiggemann, 2005).

The use of digital image manipulation has also become widespread in the advertising industry. Models with perceived normal body types can be altered to fit an extreme marketing concept, by adding muscle mass, altering facial structure, or cropping body lines and contours. The norm becomes abnormal, but the object of desire. The latter has been referred to as normative discontent in terms of women feeling inherently dissatisfied with some aspect of their body (Tiggemann, 2005; Tiggemann & Slater, 2004) and likely extends to males as well (Baghurst et al., 2006; Leone et al., 2011).

Training people at young ages to deconstruct media messages (referred to as media literacy), in order to view them as the driving impetus for the advertisement often helps limit negative reactions and behaviors. Resiliency training also may help curtail the negative influence of various media messages and marketing strategies (Lubans et al., 2016; Masten, Best & Garmezy, 1990). What is socially acceptable is constantly being redefined as culture evolves and redefines itself. Therefore, a consistent system to evaluate media messages will help people better understand social patterns and make healthier choices.

Eating disorders in males

In this section, specific eating disorders in males are explored such as under-eating, anorexia nervosa, and bulimia nervosa.

Under-eating disorders

Although much less common in males, under-eating disorders (e.g. anorexia nervosa and potentially bulimia nervosa) do occur and likely at higher than expected rates due to under-reporting. In fact, a recent report suggests common stereotypes concerning eating disorders have led to marked disparities in diagnoses in males (Sonneville & Lipson, 2018). In their study, females were five times more likely to be diagnosed with an eating disorder and were subsequently more likely to receive help. Under-eating disorders are less about weight and more about control of one's body and environment. Eating disorders focusing on caloric restriction generally stem from a psychological impulse to assert control over one's life and body. An obsession usually develops in the person's psyche followed by the compulsion to address their obsessional thought patterns. These compulsions usually take the form of controlling what one chooses to consume (Anderson, Cohn & Holbrook, 2000; Dakanalis et al., 2013).

Anorexia nervosa

Causes of anorexia nervosa

A single cause of anorexia nervosa (AN) has not been established, rather a confluence of genetic, nutritional, social, environmental, psychobehavioral, and neurobiological influences likely underpin the disorder (Dakanalis et al., 2013). As with any psychiatric disorder, specific criteria need to be met prior to a formal diagnosis of the condition. Occurrence of AN may be due to a genetic predisposition toward clinical depression and other genes that control eating regulation, emotions, and resultant eating behaviors (Thornton, Mazzeo, & Bulik, 2010).

Social factors contributing to AN are numerous and varied. The social environment and context in which a person resides often guides their perception of themselves, which may affect their eating attitudes and behaviors (Thornton et al., 2010). Rates of AN are highest among wealthy to middle class, Caucasian, females; however, rates have been calculated for men as well, accounting for up to 10% of the population with, again, the former statistic likely under-reported (Sonneville & Lipson, 2018). It has been postulated that men may experience a double hit with an eating disorder; first due to the actual issues with the disease and comorbidities and second, the social stigma attached to having what is commonly viewed as a female disease. Activities that focus on body aesthetic and weight limitations, such as dancing, wrestling, running, and rowing among others often have higher prevalence of AN (Sonneville & Lipson, 2018), although any sport or exercise participation can provide a venue for AN-related behaviors. Clearly, social and environmental factors play a key role in the development of AN.

Most people with AN overestimate their body size and their perceptions of how others view them. Recall from the previous sections that many males often *underestimate* their body size and levels of muscularity, often desiring more lean body mass. These cognitive processing issues manifest in distorted views of the body and can result in negative behaviors (e.g., excessive exercise, caloric restriction, purging) (Dakanalis et al., 2013; Sonneville & Lipson, 2018).

At risk populations

Research indicates that up to 10% of males suffer from AN with most research only conducted with Westernized industrial culture; therefore, incidence and prevalence may not be generalizable to the overall population (Sonneville & Lipson, 2018). Many people with AN also report a past or current history of sexual abuse (Steinhausen, 2002; Thornton et al., 2010). Adolescents account for nearly 40% of all reported clinical cases. Overall, populations that value restraint, aesthetics, and anti-fat attitudes tend to see higher incidence and overall prevalence of AN, males notwithstanding as previously discussed in the context of an image-conscious society (Steinhausen, 2002).

Bulimia nervosa

Causes of bulimia nervosa

Bulimia nervosa (BN) is a *DSM-V* classified eating disorder (American Psychiatric Association, 2013). Similar to AN, causes of BN are likely to be multifactorial. Depression and anxiety disorders often are associated with bulimia. Unlike AN, BN is primarily characterized by a series of food binges followed by guilt and shame resulting in efforts to purge the system. Most experts agree that BN is likely the result of psychological issues surrounding control in one's life. Using food and other unhealthy purging practices (e.g., laxatives, diuretics, vomiting, medications) helps the person with BN assert control over their emotional issues. Binging and purging becomes an addictive pattern where the binge creates the sense of guilt from the loss of control over eating habits, followed by the purging process, allowing the person to regain their lost sense of self-control. Social climate and physical activities (gymnasts, wrestlers, dancers, cheerleading) that stress eating control and weight management often see a higher prevalence of BN in both females and males (Ricciardelli, 2015).

At risk populations

BN is more likely to be seen in females than in males. Prevalence statistics suggest rates as low as 0.1% in males to 2.1% and 0.3% to 7.3% in females. These data, however, only reflect those people in treatment facilities or with a formal diagnosis of BN. Many people may practice BN-type behaviors, but are not formally diagnosed with the condition, again with males likely under-reported/under-diagnosed (Ricciardelli, 2015; Sonneville & Lipson, 2018).

Signs and symptoms of bulimia nervosa

Tell-tale signs and symptoms of BN include binges with food, which may have caloric consumption as high as 15,000 kcals in one sitting followed by the use of various methods to purge the food from the body (American Psychiatric Association, 2013). People with bulimia often look normal in terms of weight; therefore, intervention and diagnosis may present a particular challenge. There also exists a non-purge type of bulimia, which is less common (6–8% of cases) where the individual adopts excessive exercise patterns to purge calories or they may engage in a prolonged fast before or after a binge episode; recent evidence suggests this form of BN may be more prevalent in males than once thought (Ricciardelli, 2015). In particular, men who exhibit higher levels of anger may be more prone to BN and related disordered eating patterns (Penas-Lledo, Fernandez, & Waller, 2004). Abnormal attitudes toward food and eating, such as hoarding food, eating only one type of food, and any other abnormal eating practice may warrant further questioning from a qualified health care professional (American Psychiatric Association, 2013; Ricciardelli, 2015).

Overeating disorder and compulsive eating disorder

Signs and symptoms of compulsive eating disorder

Compulsive overeating is different than simply consuming greater quantities of food. A loss of control followed by guilt and/or shame often results. Unlike BN, people with compulsions to overeat do not attempt to purge the food from the body. Binge eating is a closely connected disorder where a massive amount of food and calories are consumed at one sitting or period of time (American Psychiatric Association, 2013). The latter also may be conflated with boys and men having healthy appetites, which is consistent with endorsement of masculine ideology (Connell & Messerschmidt, 2005; Leone, 2012).

Eating to the point of discomfort is not uncommon with compulsive overeaters in addition to consuming food very rapidly. Constant thoughts, talk, and preoccupation with food underpins compulsive eating behavior. Grazing or eating smaller portions throughout the day likely add up to high caloric values with the compulsion. Unlike the recommended six meals per day to optimize metabolism, persons with compulsive overeating tendencies do not plan their food consumption, but rather, engage in continuous eating throughout the day (American Psychiatric Association, 2013).

At risk populations

Any person can overeat and it is often situation dependent (i.e., holidays, vacations, etc.). What distinguishes compulsive overeating and binge eating from occasional over-indulgence is the consistency by which it manifests itself daily. Both men and women are prone to compulsive eating, but there is likely to be a strong emotional disturbance corresponding with the disorder. Those who are depressed or suffer from anxiety disorders may react by consuming food as a form of comfort. Persons with low levels of self-esteem and self-efficacy may also be prone to overeating. Last, victims of sexual abuse also may be at risk for compulsive and overeating disorders (American Psychiatric Association, 2013).

Body dysmorphic disorder

Phillips (1998) defines body dysmorphic disorder (BDD) as having three qualities: (1) pre-occupation with an imagined defect in appearance; if a slight physical anomaly is present, the person's concern is markedly excessive; (2) preoccupation causes clinically significant distress or impairment in social, occupational, or other important areas; and, (3) the pre-occupation is not better accounted for by another mental disorder. Additionally, BDD is a subcategory of obsessive–compulsive disorder (OCD) and part of the general spectrum disorders classification system (American Psychiatric Association, 2013). Often emerging in adolescence, the defining feature of BDD versus simply being dissatisfied with a part of one's body is the preoccupying and obsessive nature of it. Regardless of whether there is even a defect at all, it becomes real for the person experiencing BDD (Phillips, 1998).

Body image has been researched as a key component in social anxiety disorders and lower levels of social self-esteem (Cash, 2004; Grogan, 2016). Phillips (1998) discussed BDD as a consequence of a distorted body image. Given such a long history of body image research, body image disturbance in BDD is under-studied and warrants further research on its impact on global self-esteem and body image in general, particularly in males. For example, Leone et al. (2015) found that men who scored higher on muscle dysmorphia indices also scored higher on emotional restraint, specifically alexithymia (inability to identify and recognize emotions). The next section briefly outlines muscle dysmorphia, a sub-clinical category of body dysmorphia.

Muscle dysmorphia

Muscle dysmorphia (MD) (also referred to as reverse anorexia and bigorexia) was originally described by Pope, Katz, and Hudson (1993). Pope, Phillips, et al. state:

> Muscle dysmorphia is a specific type of BDD … the general category of BDD refers to all types of serious unfounded body image concerns. Muscle dysmorphia is a form of BDD in which muscularity, as opposed to some other aspect of the body, becomes the focus.
>
> (2000, p. 87)

Causes of MD most likely include a variety of factors ranging from sociocultural influences to genetic factors (Cerea, Bottesi, Pacelli, Paoli, & Ghisi, 2018; Pope et al., 1993). Body esteem is a key measure and component of MD (Cerea et al., 2018). Unlike other disorders, such as AN and BN, identification, diagnosis, and treatment of MD presents a challenge to the practitioner (Leone, Sedory, & Gray, 2005). This latter point may be due to the fact that people with MD often are perceived and perceive themselves to be healthy. Behaviors and attitudes often become overt to family and friends but the person experiencing MD remains oblivious.

Although not formally categorized as a *DSM-V* disorder, several researchers have proposed diagnostic criteria for MD, which is now included as a subtype of BDD (American Psychiatric Association, 2013; Murray, Rieger, Touyz, & De la Garza Garcia, 2010). When viewed as a body image disorder rather than a collection of psychiatric and behavioral oddities, MD becomes a window by which today's evolving ideals of beauty, particularly of the male body, can be seen. Although females also are susceptible to the disorder, data suggest males are more commonly affected (Cerea et al., 2018). From a traditional perspective, masculinity and muscle have defined the measure of a man (Baghurst et al., 2006; Connell & Messerschmidt, 2005). Muscle has come to symbolize health, dominance, power, strength, sexual virility, and threat, all key components in hegemonic masculinity (Baghurst et al., 2006; Connell & Messerschmidt, 2005). When there is an actual or perceived flaw with one's muscularity, obsessive thoughts and, ultimately, a concern for the body may result (Phillips, 1998; Pope, Phillips, et al., 2000). Insecurity may be a cause for the development of a hypermasculine persona or even insecurity with shifting gender roles (Connell & Messerschmidt, 2005; Pope, Phillips, et al., 2000).

Society likely plays a major role in the etiology of MD and similar body image disorders, particularly in males. Messages are broadcast that propose *real men* have big muscles and a lack thereof reflects weakness (Leone et al., 2005; Pope et al., 1993). De-masculinization often leads to a reactive approach, which may include using body-enhancing substances, such as androgenic-anabolic steroids (AAS) (Pope et al., 2017). Many males and a few females disclosed they use AAS purely for body appearance ideals rather than for athletic ideals or goals (Murray, Griffiths, Mond, Kean, & Blashill, 2016). MD, among other body image disorders, likely will continue to increase in prevalence due to media and societal influences, although actual incidence and prevalence is largely undetermined (Cerea et al., 2018; Dakanalis et al., 2013; Leone et al., 2015).

Future directions

With increased attention toward male body image and the resulting issues (i.e. drug use, risky practices, etc.), tools, programs, and trainings have been developed and implemented. Research also is in its nascent stages pertaining to males; therefore, long term success of programs and interventions is difficult to measure. The overarching goal in this line of research is establishing positive male body image; this final section will briefly detail some examples in the area of resources and tools.

Perhaps one of the most notable shifts in this line of research is movement away from body image itself and toward models of positive body image, well-being, and self-care (Halliwell, 2015). Some larger focus areas include: self-esteem, proactive coping, optimism, positive affect, self-compassion, life satisfaction, and subjective happiness, with stated goals of integrating these into therapeutic counseling approaches, programming, and interventions (Halliwell, 2015). Researchers are quick to point out that findings also need to take into account the intersections of race, gender identity, sexual orientation, and other factors concerning programming and clinical practice with men (Swami, 2015).

Working early in primary and secondary school settings also has shown promise in promoting and helping to maintain wellness and positive body image (Yager, Diedrichs, Ricciardelli, & Halliwell, 2013). College and university wellness programs also have become more inclusive in terms of psychological well-being and eating disorder awareness, in order not to stigmatize or discourage males from participating. Clinicians also may benefit by taking a more gender-sensitive approach with males, promoting more open dialogue about physical and mental health (Halliwell, 2015). A closer examination of masculine norms and cultural norms also may better inform all parties in terms of what motivates and mitigates body image dissatisfaction in males. What follows is a listing of resources pertaining to male body image and similar issues.

Useful resources

Books

Cash, T. F., & Pruzinsky, T. (Eds) (2002). *Body Image: A Handbook of Theory, Research, and Clinical Practice.* New York: Guilford Press.

Grogan, S. (2016). *Body Image:* Understanding *Body Dissatisfaction in Men, Women, and Children* (3rd ed.). London: Routledge.

Pope, H. G., Phillips, K. A., & Olivardia, R. (2000). *The Adonis Complex: The Secret Crisis of Male Body Obsession.* New York: The Free Press.

Websites

Athletes Training and Learning to Avoid Steroids (ATLAS): www.ohsu.edu/xd/education/schools/school-of-medicine/departments/clinical-departments/medicine/divisions/hpsm/research/atlas.cfm

Australian Men's Health Forum: Boy's Body Image New Digital Program: www.amhf.org.au/boys_body_image_new_digital_program_launched

National Association for Males with Eating Disorders: https://namedinc.org

The Center for Eating Disorders at Sheppard Pratt: https://eatingdisorder.org/blog/2017/06/a-focus-on-body-image-eating-disorders-in-boys-men-for-menshealthmonth/

Media

Male Body Image: A Documentary: www.youtube.com/watch?v=opV_EcA9tYs

Tough Guise 2: Violence, Manhood, and American Culture: www.jacksonkatz.com/videos/

References

American Psychiatric Association. (2013). *Diagnostic and statistical manual of mental disorders V (DSM-V)*. Washington, DC: APA Publishing.

Anderson, A. E., Cohn, L., & Holbrook, T. (2000). *Making Weight: Men's concerns with food, weight, shape and appearance*. Carlsbad, CA: Gurze Books.

Baghurst, T., Hollander, D. B., Nardella, B., & Haff, G. G. (2006). Change in sociocultural ideal male physique: An examination of past and present action figures. *Body Image, 3*(1), 87–91.

Cash, T. F. (2004). Cognitive behavioral perspectives on body image. In T. F. Cash & T. Pruzinsky (Eds.), *Body Image: A handbook of theory, research, and clinical practice* (pp. 38–46). New York: The Guilford Press.

Cerea, S., Bottesi, G., Pacelli, Q. F., Paoli, A., & Ghisi, M. (2018). Muscle dysmorphia and its associated psychological features in three groups of recreational athletes. *Scientific Reports, 8*, 8877.

Cohane, G., & Pope, H. G. (2001). Body image in boys: A review of the literature. *International Journal of Eating Disorders, 29*, 373–379.

Connell, R. W., & Messerschmidt, J. W. (2005). Hegemonic masculinity: Rethinking the concept. *Gender and Society, 19*(6), 829–859.

Dakanalis, A., Zanetti, A. M., Riva, G., Colmegna, F., Volpatao, C., Madeddu, F., & Clerici, M. (2013). Male body dissatisfaction and eating disorder symptomatology: Moderating variables among men. *Journal of Health Psychology, 20*, 80–90. https://doi.org/10.1177/1359105313499198.

Davis, C., & Cowles, M. (1991). Body image and exercise: A study of relationships and comparisons between physically active men and women. *Sex Roles, 25*, 33–44. doi: 10.1007/BF00289315

Dion, J., Hains, J., Vachon, P., Plouffe, J., Laberge, L., Perron, M., … & Leone, M. (2016). Correlates of body dissatisfaction in children. *The Journal of Pediatrics, 171*, 202–207.

Evans, R. R., Roy, J., Geiger, B. F., Werner, K. A., & Burnett, D. (2008). Ecological strategies to promote healthy body image among children. *Journal of School Health, 78*, 359–367.

Fardouly, F., & Vartarnian, L. R. (2016). Social media and body image concerns: Current research and future directions. *Current Opinion in Psychology, 9*, 1–5.

Field, A. E., Camargo Jr, C. A., Taylor, C. B., Berkey, C. S., Frazier, A. L., Gillman, M. W., & Colditz, G. A. (1999). Overweight, weight concerns, and bulimic behaviors among girls and boys. *Journal of the American Academy of Child & Adolescent Psychiatry, 38*(6), 754–760.

Franko, D. L., Fuller-Tyszkiewicz, M., Rodgers, R. F., Gattario, K. H., Frisén, A., Diedrichs, P. C., … & Shingleton, R. M. (2015). Internalization as a mediator of the relationship between conformity to masculine norms and body image attitudes and behaviors among young men in Sweden, US, UK, and Australia. *Body Image, 15*, 54–60.

Graber, J. A., Peterson, A. C., & Brooks-Gunn, J. (1996). Pubertal processes: Methods, measures and models. In J. A. Graber, A. C. Peterson, & L. Brooks-Gunn (Eds.), *Transitions Through Adolescence: Interpersonal domains and context* (pp. 25–53). Mah'wah, NJ: Erlbaum.

Grogan, S. (2016). *Body Image: Understanding body dissatisfaction in men, women, and children* (3rd ed.). London: Routledge.

Gruber, A. J., & Pope, H. G. (1999). Development of the Somatomorphic Matrix: A biaxial instrument for measuring body image in men and women. In T. S. Olds, J. Dollman, & K. I. Norton (Eds.), *Kinarthropometry VI* (pp. 217–232). Sydney: International Society for the Advancement of Kinarthropometry.

Halliwell, E. (2015). Future directions for positive body image research. *Body Image, 14,* 177–189.

Holland, G., & Tiggemann, M. (2016). A systematic review of the impact of the use of social networking sites on body image and disordered eating outcomes. *Body Image, 17,* 100–110. https://doi.org/10.1016/j.bodyim.2016.02.008.

Hrabosky, J. I., Cash, T. F., Veale, D., Neziroglu, F., Soll, E. A., Garner, D. M., ... & Phillips, K. A. (2009). Multidimensional body image comparisons among patients with eating disorders, body dysmorphic disorder, and clinical controls: A multisite study. *Body Image, 6*(3), 155–163.

Kanayama, G., Pope, H. G., & Hudson, J. I. (2001). 'Body image' drugs: A growing psychosomatic problem. *Psychotherapy and Psychosomatics, 70,* 61–65.

Leit, R. A., Gray, J. J., & Pope, H. G. (2002). The media's representation of the ideal male body: A cause for muscle dysmorphia? *International Journal of Eating Disorders,' 31,* 334–338.

Leone, J. E. (2012). *Concepts in Male Health: Perspectives across the lifespan.* San Francisco, CA: Jossey-Bass/Wiley.

Leone, J. E., Fetro, J. V., Kittleson, M. J., Welshimer, K. J., Partridge, J. A., & Robertson, S. L. (2011). Predictors of adolescents' male body image dissatisfaction: Implications for negative health practices and consequences for school health from a regionally representative sample. *Journal of School Health, 81*(4), 174–184. https://doi.org/10.1111/j.1746-1561.2010.00577.x

Leone, J. E., Sedory, E. J., & Gray, K. A. (2005). Recognition and treatment of muscle dysmorphia and related body image disorders. *Journal of Athletic Training, 40*(4), 352–357.

Leone, J. E., Wise, K. A., Mullin, E. M., Harmon, W., Moreno, N., & Drewniany, J. (2015). The effects of pubertal timing and alexithymia on symptoms of muscle dysmorphia and the drive for muscularity in men. *Psychology of Men and Masculinity, 16,* 67–77.

Lipinski, J. P., & Pope, H. G. (2002). Body ideals in young Samoan men: A comparison with men in North America and Europe. *International Journal of Men's Health, 1,* 163–171.

Lubans, D. R., Smith, J. J., Morgan, P. J., Beauchamp, M. R., Miller, A., Lonsdale, C., ... & Dally, K. (2016). Mediators of psychological well-being in adolescent boys. *Journal of Adolescent Health, 58*(2), 230–236.

Mangweth, B., Hausmann, A., Walch, T., Hotter, A., Rupp, C. I., Biebl, W., Hudson, J. I., & Pope, H. G. (2004). Body fat perception in eating-disordered men. *International Journal of Eating Disorders, 35,* 102–108.

Masten, A. S., Best, K. M., & Garmezy, N. (1990). Resilience and development: Contributions from the study of children who overcome adversity. *Development and Psychopathology, 2,* 425–444.

Murray, S. B., Griffiths, S., Mond, J. M., Kean, J., & Blashill, A. J. (2016). Anabolic steroid use and body image psychopathology in men: Delineating between appearance- versus performance-driven motivations. *Drug and Alcohol Dependence, 165,* 198–202.

Murray, S. B., Rieger, E., Touyz, S. W., & De la Garza Garcia, Y. (2010). Muscle dysmorphia and the DSM-V conundrum: Where does it belong? A review paper. *International Journal of Eating Disorders, 43*(6), 483–491.

Penas-Lledo, E., Fernandez, J., & Waller, G. (2004). Association of anger with bulimic and other impulsive behaviours among non-clinical women and men. *European Eating Disorders Review, 12*(6), 392–397.

Phillips, K. A. (1998). *The Broken Mirror: Understanding and treating body dysmorphic disorder.* New York: Oxford University Press.

Pope, H. G., Jr., Gruber, A. J., Mangweth, B., Bureau, B., Decol, C., Jouvent, R., & Hudson, J. I. (2000). Body image perception among men in three countries. *American Journal of Psychiatry, 157*(8), 1297–1301.

Pope, H. G., Katz, D. L., & Hudson, J. I. (1993). Anorexia nervosa and 'reverse anorexia nervosa' among 108 male bodybuilders. *Comprehensive Psychiatry, 34,* 406–409.

Pope, H. G., Khalsa, J. H., & Bhasin, S. (2017). Body image disorders and abuse of anabolic-androgenic steroids among men. *JAMA, 317*(1), 23–24.

Pope, H. G., Olivardia, R., Borowiecki, J. J., & Cohane, G. H. (2001). The growing commercial value of the male body: A longitudinal survey of advertising in women's magazines. *Psychotherapy and Psychosomatics, 70,* 189–192.

Pope, H. G., Phillips, K. A., & Olivardia, R. (2000). *The Adonis Complex: The secret crisis of male body obsession.* New York: The Free Press.

Ricciardelli, L. A. (2015). Eating disorders in boys and men. In T. Wade (Ed.), *Encyclopedia of Feeding and Eating Disorders.* Singapore: Springer.

Ricciardelli, L. A., & McCabe, M. P. (2001). Children's body image concerns and eating disturbance: A review of the literature. *Clinical Psychology Review, 21,* 325–344.

Sarwer, D. B., Cash, T. F., Magee, L., Williams, E. F., Thompson, J. K., Roehrig, M., ... & Anderson, D. A. (2005). Female college students and cosmetic surgery: An investigation of experiences, attitudes, and body image. *Plastic and Reconstructive Surgery, 115*(3), 931–938.

Sarwer, D. B., & Polonsky, H. M. (2016). Body image and body contouring procedures. *Aesthetic Surgery Journal, 36*(9), 1039–1047. https://doi.org/10.1093/asj/sjw127

Sonneville, K. R., & Lipson, S. K. (2018). Disparities in eating disorder diagnosis and treatment according to weight status, race/ethnicity, socioeconomic background, and sex among college students. *International Journal of Eating Disorders, 51*(6), 518–526.

Steinhausen, H. C. (2002). The outcome of anorexia nervosa in the 20th century. *American Journal of Psychiatry, 159,* 1284–1293.

Striegel-Moore, R. H., & Franko, D. L. (2004). Body image issues among girls and women. In T. F. Cash & T. Pruzinsky (Eds.), *Body Image: A handbook of theory, research, and clinical practice* (pp. 183–191). New York, NY: The Guilford Press.

Swami, V. (2015). Cultural influences on body size ideals. *European Psychologist, 20,* 44–51.

Thornton, L. M., Mazzeo, S. E., & Bulik, C. M. (2010). The heritability of eating disorders: Methods and current findings. In R. Adan & W. Kaye (Eds.), *Behavioral Neurobiology of Eating Disorders: Current topics in behavioral neurosciences, vol. 6* (pp. 141–156). Berlin/Heidelberg: Springer.

Tiggeman, M. (2005). Television and adolescent body image: The role of program content and viewing motivation. *Journal of Social Clinical Psychology, 24,* 361–381.

Tiggemann, M., & Slater, A. (2004). Thin ideals in music television: A source of social comparison and body dissatisfaction. *International Journal of Eating Disorders, 35,* 48–58.

Westmoreland-Corson, P., & Anderson, A. E. (2004). Body image issues among boys and men. In T. F. Cash & T. Pruzinsky (Eds.), *Body Image: A handbook of theory, research, and clinical practice* (pp. 192–199). New York, NY: The Guilford Press.

Yager, Z., Diedrichs, P. C., Ricciardelli, L., & Halliwell, E. (2013). What works in secondary schools? A systematic review of classroom-based body image programs. *Body Image, 10,* 271–281.

Part II

The body

4 Male anatomy

Michael J. Rovito and Razan Maxson

General anatomy

General overview of male urogenital anatomy

One of the most famous illustrations including the male anatomy is, arguably, Da Vinci's 'Vitruvian Man' (see Figure 4.1).

A masterpiece of the blending of humans, nature, and mathematics, this drawing is a foundation to understanding the notions of proportion and symmetry of the human body, much akin to the symmetry of the universe. Cornerstone to this drawing is the male genitalia, just below the nexus of the piece, the navel. There's nothing sexualized about the penis and testicles here. There is nothing vulgar. It is a man, inclusive of his genitalia, portrayed naturally. This is a prime example of how the male form, when placed into a proper context can transcend "the indecent" and become "the appropriate."

So, what does it mean to be male? While the definition may differ from culture to culture, the scientific community usually agrees that a certain number of anatomical features make a "male" of a certain species. Human males have a genotype of XY for their 23rd pair of chromosomes, also known as the sex chromosomes. This genotype, through various processes, gives rise to the phenotype (i.e. the expression of the genes) of a man.

Generally, and we stress *generally*, human males have distinct external genitalia, consisting of (1) the penis and (2) the scrotum, and some distinct internal organs.

The penis is subdivided into three parts: (1) the root, (2) the shaft, and (3) the glans. The root of the penis, which is the part of the penis attached to the pelvis and abdominal wall, consists of two sub-parts, the crura and the bulb.

The body is the middle portion, commonly known as the shaft. The body of the penis consists of three cylindrical spaces of soft tissue. Two larger cylindrical spaces of soft tissue, called the corpora cavernosa, are located side by side and form the bulk of the penis. When they fill with blood, the penis enlarges and becomes rigid, forming an erection. The third cylindrical space of tissue, called the corpus spongiosum, surrounds the urethra, which forms the urinary passage. The glans penis is the cone-shaped end or head of the penis, which is the termination of the corpus spongiosum. The small ridge that separates the glans penis from the shaft/body of the penis is called the corona.

The scrotum is the fleshy sack that holds the other external portion of the male genitalia: (1) testicles, (2) epididymis, (3) vas deferens, and (4) spermatic cords. The testicles are suspended within the scrotum via the spermatic cords. They are suspended unevenly, usually with the left testicle positioned lower than the right. This is normal and a method the body adopted to prevent crowding. It is within these testicles that sperm and testosterone are produced in males. It is important as a male to become familiar with this portion of

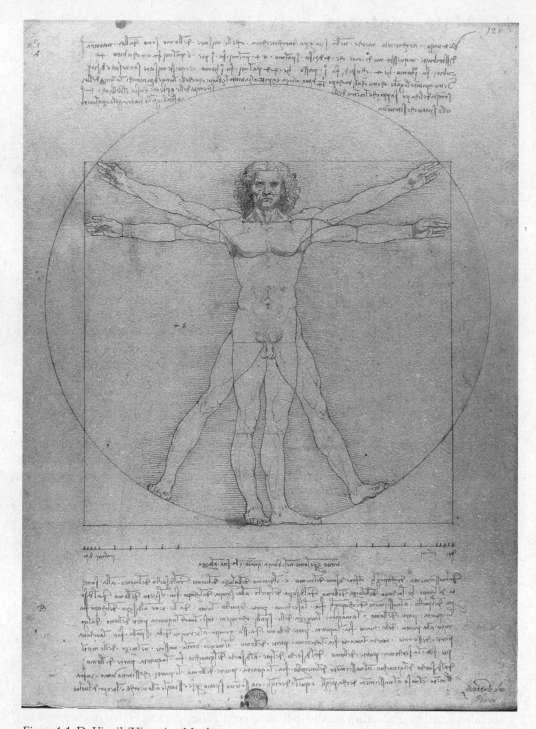

Figure 4.1 Da Vinci's 'Vitruvian Man'.

Source: This image is available at https://commons.wikimedia.org/wiki/File:Vitruvian.jpg.

the male anatomy because abnormalities can be spotted/felt with relative ease due to the external nature of the male gonads. Later in the chapter we will discuss testicular self-examination (TSE), a somewhat controversial topic in the medical community as of this writing.

The epididymis transports sperm from the testicles to the vas deferens. The vas deferens are ducts that then carry the sperm to ejaculatory ducts for the process of ejaculation. The epididymis is coiled around the back of both testicles. Each one can reach a length of 20+ feet if stretched out in a straight line. The vas deferens, which actually forms the spermatic cord, is also coiled (partially, however) and can run nearly a foot long.

The prostate (see Figure 4.2) is about the size of an apricot or a shelled walnut. It's a muscular gland responsible for producing a fluid in which semen lives and travels when ejaculated from the testicles out through the urethra. During ejaculation, the prostate closes the bladder off from the urethra to prevent the mixing of urine and semen.

Part of having the male gonads (testes) is the production of testosterone and its effects on the body. These more generalized effects are known as the secondary male characteristics. They include features that you are probably already picturing: increased size, weight, brain size, hair follicles, and bone differences when compared to females. With regard to the differences between males and females, perhaps it is best if we start from the very beginning … in the womb.

In-utero development: differentiation and fetal development

In the early stages of development in the womb, a fetus has no anatomic or hormonal sex, only a karyotype. This means that the sex chromosome being XX or XY distinguishes a male fetus from a female one. Specific genes then induce gonadal differences, which go on to produce hormonal differences that, in turn, cause anatomic differences. See Table 4.1 for a brief list of the changes that happen once the fetus starts to differentiate.

As you can see, there is both overlap in parts that "get used" in development and differences in what degrades. During these changes, and subsequent development, there are plenty of steps in which something could go wrong. These problems in development can lead to some of the conditions that will be briefly covered later in the chapter.

General anatomical differences between males and females

As is the theme throughout this chapter, to go into exhaustive explanations for any one of these topics would not serve its purpose, which is, again, to give you some brief background information for you to take a deeper dive whenever appropriate. Therefore, the following will present only the very basics of anatomical differences between males and females.

The authors want to acknowledge individuals who are born intersex, or born with the sex characteristics of a binary male/female classification. These differences may include genitals, gonads, and other chromosomal expressions. Although this is the extent to which this topic will be discussed in this chapter, there is a much larger conversation in the literature on the genesis of such expressions, as well as contemporary issues of intersex inclusion, discrimination against intersexed individuals, and health concerns experienced by this group. Reisner et al.'s (2016) review of the global health burden among this population is a great place to begin if you choose to learn more about the topic.

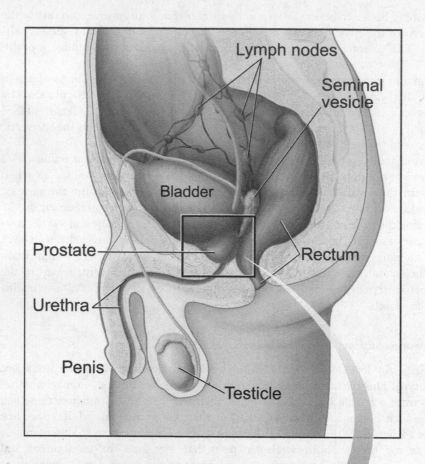

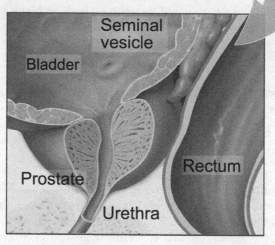

National Cancer Institute

Figure 4.2 Cross-section of male anatomy.
Source: National Cancer Institute; created by Alan Hoofring (illustrator).

Table 4.1 A comparison of male and female genetic expression, gonadal differences, and physical differentiation

Feminization	⬅ *Undifferentiated fetus* ➡	Masculinization
Ovaries	Bipotential gonads	Testes
Degrade	Wolffian ducts	Epididymis, vas deferens, seminal vesicles
Oviducts and uterus	Mullerian ducts	*Degrade*
Urinary bladder, urethra, uterus, vagina	Cloaca	Urinary bladder, urethra

Source: Created by the chapter authors.

Generally, males and females differ anatomically due to the expression, production, and presence of several hormones and chemicals. The most prominent hormones are estrogens and androgens, and the amount of each of these will vary in each person's body. Generally, although both are present in both males and females, males produce and present with more androgen while females produce and present with more estrogen. This becomes most obvious during puberty when testicles begin to produce enhanced levels of testosterone and the ovaries begin to produce enhanced levels of estradiol. Specifically, it's not so much about the total amount of either in the blood individually, but the ratio of one to the other in the bloodstream (Dluzen, 2005; Goymann & Wingfield, 2014). For example, males have approximately a 3:1 ratio of testosterone to estradiol, and women have approximately a 1:1 ratio. Males produce more than 20 times more testosterone than females, but females convert approximately 200 times the amount of testosterone to estrogens than males do.

Having more testosterone in the bloodstream is associated with, but not limited to, increased sex drive, the growth of body hair on face, neck, and rest of body, sperm production, muscle mass growth and strength, and prostate growth. Having more estrogens in the bloodstream is associated with, but not limited to, stimulation of breast development and future milk production, the growth and maturation of the uterus, ovaries, and vagina, and stimulation of the start of a female's menstrual cycle. It doesn't take too much variation in testosterone or estrogens to cause these physical changes in an individual.

Pertaining to male-specific reproductive organs and how they differ from females, most people are aware that a male usually is born with a penis, testicles, and a prostate, including all the additional sub-anatomies that make up any one of these (i.e. the epididymis of a testicle, the vas deferens, the crura of a penis, etc.). A female, in contrast, does not have any of these organs. They are born usually with ovaries, fallopian tubes, a cervix, and a vagina. Again, this is stated within the scope of generality. There are other, more specific, differences between males and females, including brain physicality (Brizendine, 2006) and vocal anatomies (Fitch & Giedd, 1999), among others, that are not covered here.

Congenital male-specific health concerns

There are many health concerns that affect male anatomy uniquely. Unsurprisingly, the most distinguishing ones are seen within urogenital systems. The following section highlights current health and wellness trends among males. This is a short list of the more prevalent issues males face during development.

Hypospadias

A common birth defect in males is hypospadias. This defect occurs during in-utero development during weeks 8–14 of pregnancy and occurs in one out of every 200 males (Mayo Clinic, 2018a). Males born with this defect have a urethra that opens not at the tip of the penis, as is usual, but anywhere from where the penis and scrotum meet, all along the shaft, and near the head of the penis. There are, generally, three major types of hypospadias: (1) glanural (i.e. distal), (2) coronal, and (3) penile shaft. There is a fourth type, which is the least common and most serious kind. It's called perineal hypospadias. This is when the opening sets behind the scrotum. Surgery, sometimes multistage, is required to correct the defect otherwise issues with urination and copulation can occur.

Chordee

Often seen with cases of hypospadias, chordee is a condition in which the penis has excessive ventral (downward) curvature. It can be caused by circumcision, a topic that is covered later in this chapter. Surgery is required to repair chordee and is often done before correcting hypospadias, if present. Often, this disorder is confused with Peyronie's disease. However, Peyronie's disease is a curvature of the penis that is usually the result of some type of injury during adulthood.

Cryptorchidism

Cryptorchidism is also known as undescended testicle. With a rising prevalence of up to 9% of male newborns (Virtanen & Toppari, 2007), cryptorchidism has become a major male health issue; not so much for the immediate lack of a testicle in the scrotum at the time of diagnosis, but because of the complications in later life (Kinkade, 1999). The undescended testicle being sequestered in the adverse intra-abdominal environment makes it susceptible to mutagenic changes. In fact, cryptorchidism is one of the most significant established risk factors for the development of testicular cancer (TCa) and infertility in adulthood, even with surgical correction.

Swyer syndrome

Swyer syndrome is also known as XY gonadal dysgenesis (when your genotype doesn't match your phenotype). This disorder occurs in one out of every 80,000 male births. Males with Swyer syndrome present externally as female. Internally they develop a uterus and oviducts but lack functional gonads, neither testes nor ovaries, which means their bipotential gonads never differentiated. This undifferentiated tissue can become cancerous and is usually removed early in life. Hormone replacement therapy can be used in adolescence to induce development of secondary female characteristics and promote menstruation. These individuals, though XY in genotype, can become pregnant via donated egg/embryo.

Early childhood development health concerns

Once the male baby is born and makes it past any immediate concerns, such as those mentioned previously, there is a whole new batch of potential health issues and decisions that parents need to be aware of. Alongside having to deal with a young mind exploring and discovering their body, there is also the eventual transition of an adolescent male into puberty and sexual maturity. At some point during this period in a male's life a major decision, and one that has become more and more controversial, needs to be made and that decision is whether to circumcise.

Circumcision

What is it? If you are reading this in a part of the world where the practice is not commonplace you may not even be aware that young males, or their parents, in other countries find themselves needing to make this decision. You may not even be aware of what the procedure is, or the reasons why some people do it. Circumcision is, in short, the surgical removal of the foreskin of the penis. Circumcision, in all its forms, has been practiced, banned and practiced again by a variety of cultures. It is a tradition that has multiple origins and has been observed throughout these different cultures around the world, stretching back thousands of years. The amount of foreskin removed varies depending on the culture and time-period of the practice. Subsequently, the reasons for circumcision were, and are, as different as the people who practiced it.

A male could be circumcised as a symbolic transition to manhood, such as with the Maasai people in Kenya or Tanzania. A boy in a Maasai tribe would eagerly await his opportunity to partake in this rite of passage and prove that he is worthy of being elevated in the eyes of his people from childhood to adulthood (Saitoti, 1988). Circumcision is also practiced as a method to help prevent sexually transmitted diseases. In fact, the World Health Organization (WHO) reports that three randomized control trials showed a 60% reduction in the risk of acquiring HIV in heterosexual males who were circumcised (WHO, 2007).

Not all circumcision, however, was/is practiced for what could be considered positive reasons. It has been used as a way of forcing a religion or culture onto non-consenting adults, as a way to inflict pain on a young adult male in an effort to curb sexual appetites/deterrent against masturbation (Kellogg, 1882), or even as a symbolic commitment to a covenant with a supreme being (Posner, 2018). Though circumcision rates are on the decline in the United States (Centers for Disease Control and Prevention, 2011), as with many parts of the world, there are still certain populations, followers of the Jewish and Muslim faith, for example, that have near 99% circumcision rates (Morris et al., 2016). As such, this will remain a topic with a growing body of data to keep an eye on. Perhaps the next shift in recommendations from the WHO or similar organizations, and therefore future prevalence rates, is on the horizon.

Other health concerns, issues, and topics

Prostate cancer

The basics

The most common type of cancer in males is prostate cancer (PCa) (Mayo Clinic, 2018b). Culp, Soerjomataram, Efstathiou, Bray, and Jemal (2020) indicated that the United States, Northern/Western Europe, Australia/New Zealand, and the Caribbean have the highest incidence rates of PCa while sub-Saharan Africa, portions of Southeast Asia, the former

Soviet Union, and the Caribbean have the highest mortality rates of the disease. PCa is a slow-growing cancer (most times), but there can be more aggressive cases, particularly seen among younger males. Usually, PCa presents in middle-aged to older males (55+ years of age) cases can be seen in even younger populations (35–45 years of age), though this is rare.

If PCa is detected in its early stages where it is confined to the prostate itself and not metastasized, no serious harm is experienced. There are some rarer instances of adverse reactions to treatment, but the disease itself, in almost every situation, when detected and treated in the early stages, will have a fantastic prognosis. The later the stage of detection and treatment, the lower the chances of successful outcomes, which is what is most common among less-developed societies. These outcomes are not just survivorship, but of high quality of life post treatment.

Some symptoms of the disease include persistent groin, pelvic, and/or back pain, blood in semen or urine, trouble with urinating, erectile dysfunction, and urine flow issues. However, these are seen in more advanced cases. In its infancy and early stages, usually, PCa has no obvious signs or symptoms, which contributes to concerns with screening and detection services.

Screening guidelines

When discussing screening guidelines for PCa, it is important to discuss the groups most at-risk of getting the disease, and especially those most at-risk of being diagnosed at later stages. Generally, older men (50+) that have a family history of the disease are common candidates to begin getting screened for PCa. However, there are also other factors that weigh in on when, or even if, a man should undergo screening. For example, African American males are more likely to get diagnosed at later stages and die of the disease than other ethnic/racial groups (Rogers et al., 2018). Further, there is emerging literature suggesting links between the BRCA (BReast CAncer) genes and the development of PCa (Castro, Goh, & Olmos, 2013).

Considering the above risk factors, usually a male will undergo a series of three steps during routine screening: (1) prostate-specific antigen test (PSA), (2) family history analysis, and (3) a digital rectal exam (DRE). The prostate produces PSA which is found in sperm and blood. The PSA test is a simple blood test used primarily to detect the amount of PSA in the bloodstream. As males age, their prostate grows, and as a result, secretes more PSA. Males with PCa may see elevated levels of PSA in the blood, but not all males with elevated levels of PSA have PCa.

There are issues, though, regarding PCa screening, particularly regarding the use of PSA. One of the main reasons for this is the existence of elevated PSA cases not related to PCa manifestation. Kearns et al. (2018) outline the reasons why the United States Preventive Services Task Force (USPSTF) granted it a "D" rating, which means they recommend against its use in the clinic. Although "treatment as usual" would consist of the PSA test, it is used in tandem with a complete historical analysis of PCa in the family, as well as a DRE. A DRE is when a physician palpates the prostate through the anus and rectum for abnormalities.

There have been unintended consequences, though. For example, Ahlering et al. (2019), among others, point to the idea that although PCa has decreased in overall incidence among certain communities, it is not due to the disease ceasing to exist, but rather a lack of action on capturing existing, undiagnosed cases. In other words, PCa still existed, they just weren't capturing all the cases out there.

Testicular cancer

The basics

Testicular cancer (TCa) is the most prevalent form of cancer among men aged 15–35 (Adams, Rovito, & Craycraft, 2018), if you take into consideration domestic rates. Global risk estimates suggest that the ages of 18–44 years of age are the prime years of TCa occurrence. Global regions with the highest incidence of the disease include Northern/ Western Europe, the United States, and Australia/New Zealand. Sub-Saharan Africa has the lowest rates. The groups with the highest rates across all regions are those males who are of Scandinavian descent.

TCa occurs, of course, in the testicles. Some symptoms include heaviness in the groin, persistent back pain, palpable mass/lump on the testicles, and tenderness/pain/discomfort in the testicles (Mayo Clinic, 2018c). TCa usually occurs in one testicle but can affect the other in some rare cases. Risk factors of the disease include family history, your age (usually teenagers into middle-aged adults), race (mostly Caucasians are affected), and cryptorchidism. However, there has been a lack of hard evidence linking any causal factors to the disease. Prevention of the disease, therefore, is difficult.

TCa is a fast-growing cancer, which is why early detection is of utmost importance to overall survival (McGilligan, McClenahan, & Adamson, 2009). The lack of TCa information dissemination limits prevention behaviors, contributing to a 50% diagnosis rate of metastatis from the testes (Trumbo, 2004).

Screening guidelines

Testicular examination, either completed by a physician or by the male himself (i.e. TSE), is the prominent form of screening for TCa. However, there's contention among health professionals whether screening for TCa successfully reduces mortality from the disease as the treatment is so effective. Essentially, even at later stages, full recovery is not just possible, but probable. In early stages, the five-year survival rate of TCa is near 100%. In later stages, that figure dips into the 70–80% range. Therefore, opponents of TSE claim there is no point conducting screening because the cure rate is so high. They also claim that males experience undue anxiety if they experience a false positive. However, there's a lack of evidence to back up this claim. Any anxiety experienced because of false-positive detections can easily be justified by the prevention of late-stage diagnosis and the complications associated with invasive treatment, including anxiety, secondary malignancies, and decreased quality of life, among others.

Rovito, Leone, and Cavayero (2018) argued that expanding TSE beyond exclusively TCa detection can provide an opportunity to detect other noncancerous testicular abnormalities, such as varicocele, hydrocele, epididymitis, and orchitis, among others. Yet, the USPSTF grants a "D" rating for recommending TSE, which means that they recommend against performing the behavior (Rovito, Manjelievskaia, Leone, Lutz, & Nangia, 2016). However, due to the lack of evidence claiming TSE causes more harm than benefit, the behavior should at least be practiced by those males with a history of risk factors, like cryptorchidism, family history, and microlithiasis (the formation of calcium clusters in the testicles), among others.

Reaching males

The field of men's health, at least in the public health sector, is rooted squarely in promotion of agency (i.e. ability to produce desired health outcomes), knowledge, and awareness. Generally, the field is interested in engaging males and empowering them to make sound, informed decisions pertaining to their health and wellbeing. Engaging and/ or re-engaging males, however, can be a daunting task. There's not enough room in this book, let alone this one chapter, to thoroughly discuss innovative ways to get males more actively engaged with their health and wellbeing. Therefore, we provide an outline of some umbrella concepts that have shown some influence on the health and wellbeing of boys and men. This section provides you some tools that you may find useful when searching for information regarding the health and wellbeing of the male anatomy.

Interpersonal and institutional barriers

Awareness and knowledge of a disease or health issue tends to be the primary reason why males fail to navigate the healthcare system when faced with a particular concern (Garcia, Ptak, Stelzer, Harwood, & Brady, 2014). Evans, Frank, Oliffe, and Gregory (2011) also discuss the role of masculinity serving as a barrier to healthcare navigation as it pertains to fear, stigma, embarrassment, and loss of social status when thinking about, or trying to obtain, assistance with some health concern. Males have been conforming to social norms of masculinity since the dawn of time, which has potentially deadly results. That sounds a bit alarming, but when males fail to want to receive treatment for a health issue despite obvious and very serious persistent symptoms over prolonged periods of time (e.g. blood in urine or stool), prognoses tend to be less than ideal. Many cases of prostate cancer turn out deadly when they didn't have to be.

In addition to interpersonal barriers, men also face institutional barriers when attempting to navigate the healthcare system. These can range from a lack of cultural competency when discussing male-specific health concerns, confidentiality concerns, and perceived judgment from healthcare workers, among others (Alsan & Wanamaker, 2017; Balfe & Brugha, 2009; Gornick, 2008; Lanier & Sutton, 2013). Even if a male does circumnavigate his own internal barriers to seeking healthcare, institutional barriers may prevent him from getting the attention he needs.

Targeted interventions

Pringle et al. (2014) suggest that often it's not the fault of males when they show a disinterest in health or a lack of willingness to engage the healthcare system. Many times, in fact, it's the way we are going about discussing it with them or promoting the system to them. The forum, they suggest, is out of sync with how males would like to consume healthcare. Interventions aimed at promoting health and wellness to males are flawed in two primary ways: (1) targeted messages are not created specifically for males or (2) targeted messages speak to a small group of males.

For example, it may be disadvantageous for the field of men's health to make any progress if we continue to approach males as if they all respond to football analogies, "boys will be boys" mentalities, fist-bumping, and thrill-seeking, rife with references to extreme sports, competition, and the most toxic of stereotypical masculine traits, including the hypersexualized, hyperaggressive male. Taglines like "man up" or "suck it up" are consistently employed to promote action, or we make references to male genitalia in a joking manner to make light of the situation regarding, usually, male cancers. These phrases and "jokes" promote the hegemonic masculine ideal which restricts the socially acceptable spectrum of emotions for men to things such as anger and stoic confidence (Donaldson, 1993). Most, if not all, mass-mediated TCa awareness campaigns, for example, use the word "balls," "nuts," "nads," or some other slang term to reference testicles. Not only is this anatomization of manhood exclusionary, not all men have testicles, it is also likely that many men will react negatively to such reductive language; people are not their genitals.

What's next?

Much work needs to be done, ranging from the government and policy level down to the patient–provider relationship. At the global and national levels, creating Offices of Men's Health or developing male-specific policies would be a great first step. Baker and Brown's (2018) critique of the current state of global health policies involving men and boys is a wonderful place to start for any burgeoning student of the field. At the patient–provider level, more work needs to be done connecting men with holistic health services at the point of contact, such as with men's health clinics and community health centers.

But, this is another topic for another day. For now, remember, male anatomy can bring about serious health concerns. We need to approach the topic, not with hesitation or a tongue-in-cheek approach, but with an open mind and a willingness to have an honest and open conversation. There are many great resources available to navigate this issue. We include some of these sources for you to start diving into that rabbit hole to get more informed on the topic.

Vignette

We leave you with a personal story from one of the author's own experience with TCa. This was a watershed moment in his life that decided for him what his passion would be for his personal and professional future. The point of including this personal account is to promote active learning among males. They must know and understand their own anatomy. Only when males are informed about their body and what complications can occur as they age can we truly be effective in improving both the quantity and quality of years lived.

In his own words

It's a very odd feeling when you discover a lump in/on your body. I usually describe to people that it feels like a sense of disbelief with a hint of "are you kidding me?" I found a lump on my left testicle when I was 17 years old. As soon as I felt it, I thought it was cancer. I really didn't know too much about my health besides that I should eat and exercise healthily and that I probably shouldn't smoke cigarettes with my friends. But, in a sense, I was innocently ignorant of what I should know and what I should be doing. I was hesitant to let anyone know what I had found and I had very limited options to figure out what this lump was. A 17-year-old young man usually has reservations bringing up most health concerns to anybody, particularly when it involves anything below the belt and above the thighs. I chose to keep it to myself and worry, until I found it in me to see a urologist. During the examination, which lasted about 10 seconds but felt like forever, I started to cry. Men don't cry, right? Nonsense. Men do cry. Boys do cry. I cried. I was told that I had a varicocele and that it was treatable. It was at that point I not only learned the importance to knowing my body and paying attention to my health but that it's also ok to feel vulnerable. The varicocele came back about a decade later and I underwent treatment for it again. But this time around, I was more equipped to deal with the situation. I knew I had to be more aware of my body so I can be healthier.

Additional resources

The following resources are great for further exploration of the male anatomy and related health topics.

Pop culture

1. The documentary, *Balls*, is an interesting hour-long take on testicles. It's humorous, informative, and definitely worth the watch. (www.imdb.com/title/tt5545960/?ref_=ttpl_pl_tt)
2. Vitruvian Man is more complex than meets the eye. The following resources are interesting in the sense that it's a near-perfect blending of mathematics and anatomy
   a. The film, *The Mystery of the Vitruvian Man* (www.imdb.com/title/tt1734553/)
   b. From the TED-ed video series: *Da Vinci's Vitruvian Man of Math* (www.imdb.com/title/tt5545960/?ref_=ttpl_pl_tt)

Other resources

1. *Inner Body* is an interactive web-based platform from which you can learn all about the different parts of the male anatomy. (www.innerbody.com/image/repmov.html)
2. The Australian government has some interesting resources to learn more about male anatomy and reproductive health. There are some good graphics, videos, and other information that can help you establish your own knowledge base or help you create lessons to assist others in understanding this topic. https://gdhr.wa.gov.au/-/reproduction-and-anatomy

References

Adams, W. B., Rovito, M. J., & Craycraft, M. (2018). The connection between testicular cancer, minority males, and Planned Parenthood. *American Journal of Men's Health, 12*(5), 1774–1783.

Ahlering, T., Huynh, L. M., Kaler, K. S., Williams, S., Osann, K., Joseph, J., … & Patel, V. (2019). Unintended consequences of decreased PSA-based prostate cancer screening. *World Journal of Urology, 37*(3), 489–496.

Alsan, M., & Wanamaker, M. (2017). Tuskegee and the health of black men. *The Quarterly Journal of Economics, 133*(1), 407–455.

Baker, P., & Brown, A. (2018). Men's health: time for a policy response. *International Journal of Men's Social and Community Health, 1*(SP1), e1–e5.

Balfe, M., & Brugha, R. (2009). What prompts young adults in Ireland to attend health services for STI testing? *BMC Public Health, 9*(1), 31.

Brizendine, L. (2006). *The Female Brain.* Broadway Books.

Castro, E., Goh, C., & Olmos, D. (2013). Germline BRCA mutations are associated with higher risk of nodal involvement, distant metastasis, and poor survival outcomes in prostate cancer. *Journal of Clinical Oncology, 31*(14), 1748.

Centers for Disease Control and Prevention. (2011, September 2). Trends in in-hospital newborn male circumcision — United States, 1999–2010. *Morbidity and Mortality Weekly Report, 60*(34), 1167. Retrieved from www.cdc.gov/mmwr/pdf/wk/mm6034.pdf

Culp, M. B., Soerjomataram, I., Efstathiou, J. A., Bray, F., & Jemal, A. (2020). Recent global patterns in prostate cancer incidence and mortality rates. *European Urology, 77*(1), 38–52.

Dluzen, D. E. (2005). Estrogen, testosterone, and gender differences. *Endocrine, 27*(3), 259–267.

Donaldson, M. (1993). What is hegemonic masculinity? *Theory and Society, 22*(5), 643–657.

Evans, J., Frank, B., Oliffe, J. L., & Gregory, D. (2011). Health, illness, men and masculinities (HIMM): a theoretical framework for understanding men and their health. *Journal of Men's Health, 8*(1), 7–15.

Fitch, W. T., & Giedd, J. (1999). Morphology and development of the human vocal tract: a study using magnetic resonance imaging. *The Journal of the Acoustical Society of America, 106*(3), 1511–1522.

Garcia, C. M., Ptak, S. J., Stelzer, E. B., Harwood, E. M., & Brady, S. S. (2014). "I connect with the ringleader:" Health professionals' perspectives on promoting the sexual health of adolescent males. *Research in Nursing & Health, 37*(6), 454–465.

Gornick, M. E. (2008). A decade of research on disparities in Medicare utilization: lessons for the health and health care of vulnerable men. *American Journal of Public Health, 98*(Supplement 1), S162–S168.

Goymann, W., & Wingfield, J. C. (2014). Male-to-female testosterone ratios, dimorphism, and life history: what does it really tell us? *Behavioral Ecology, 25*(4), 685–699.

Kearns, J. T., Holt, S. K., Wright, J. L., Lin, D. W., Lange, P. H., & Gore, J. L. (2018). PSA screening, prostate biopsy, and treatment of prostate cancer in the years surrounding the USPSTF recommendation against prostate cancer screening. *Cancer, 124*(13), 2733–2739.

Kellogg, J. H. (1882). Plain Facts for Old and Young. IF Segner.

Kinkade, S. (1999) Testicular cancer. *American Family Physician, 59*(9), 2539–2544.

Lanier, Y., & Sutton, M. Y. (2013). Reframing the context of preventive health care services and prevention of HIV and other sexually transmitted infections for young men: new opportunities to reduce racial/ethnic sexual health disparities. *American Journal of Public Health, 103*(2), 262–269.

Mayo Clinic. (2018a). *Hypospadias.* Retrieved from www.mayoclinic.org/diseases-conditions/hypospadias/symptoms-causes/syc-20355148

Mayo Clinic (2018b). *Prostate cancer.* Retrieved from www.mayoclinic.org/diseases-conditions/prostate-cancer/symptoms-causes/syc-20353087

Mayo Clinic (2018c). *Testicular cancer.* Retrieved from www.mayoclinic.org/diseases-conditions/testicular-cancer-care/symptoms-causes/syc-20352986

McGilligan, C., McClenahan, C., & Adamson, G. (2009). Attitudes and intentions to performing testicular self-examination: utilizing an extended theory of planned behavior. *Journal of Adolescent Health, 44,* 404–406.

Morris, B. J., Wamai, R. G., Henebeng, E. B., Tobian, A. A., Klausner, J. D., Banerjee, J., & Hankins, C. A. (2016). Estimation of country-specific and global prevalence of male circumcision. *Population Health Metrics, 14*(1), 4.

Posner, M. (2018). *20 facts about Judaism that everyone should know.* Retrieved from www.chabad.org/library/article_cdo/aid/4160682/jewish/20-Facts-About-Jewish-Circumcision-Everyone-Should-Know.htm

Pringle, A., Smolinsky, S., McKenna, J., Robertson, S., Daly-Smith, A., & White, A. (2014). Health improvement for men and hard-to-engage-men delivered in English Premier League football clubs. *Health Education Research, 29*(3), 503–520.

Reisner, S. L., Poteat, T., Keatley, J., Cabral, M., Mothopeng, T., Dunham, E., … & Baral, S. D. (2016). Global health burden and needs of transgender populations: a review. *The Lancet, 388*(10042), 412–436.

Rogers, C. R., Rovito, M. J., Hussein, M., Obidike, O. J., Pratt, R., Alexander, M., … & Warlick, C. (2018). Attitudes toward genomic testing and prostate cancer research among Black men. *American Journal of Preventive Medicine, 55*(5), S103–S111.

Rovito, M. J., Leone, J. E., & Cavayero, C. T. (2018). "Off-label" usage of testicular self-examination (TSE): benefits beyond cancer detection. *American Journal of Men's Health, 12*(3), 505–513.

Rovito, M. J., Manjelievskaia, J., Leone, J. E., Lutz, M. J., & Nangia, A. (2016). From "D" to "I": A critique of the current United States preventive services task force recommendation for testicular cancer screening. *Preventive Medicine Reports, 3,* 361–366.

Saitoti, T. O. (1988). *The Worlds of a Maasai Warrior: An autobiography.* University of California Press.

Trumbo, C. (2004). Mass-mediated information effects on testicular self-examination among college students. *Journal of American College Health, 52*(6), 257–262.

Virtanen, H. E., & Toppari, J. (2007). Epidemiology and pathogenesis of cryptorchidism. *Human Reproduction Update, 14*(1), 49–58.

WHO. (2007). Male circumcision and HIV prevention www.who.int/hiv/pub/malecircumcision/mc_mr_21june07.pdf

5 Sexual health

Susan A. Milstein

Sexual behaviors

The word "sex" may mean different things to different people. Some people think of it only as penile-vaginal intercourse, while other people also include anal intercourse and oral sex. Due to these varying definitions, it's not always easy to get an accurate picture of what behaviors people are engaging in when you simply ask about "sex." People may choose to engage, or not engage, in sexual behaviors for a variety of reasons. These reasons can include everything from cultural and religious upbringing, to body image, to a history of sexual trauma, and sexual preferences.

Starting in 2009, researchers at Indiana University began one of the largest national surveys of sexual behaviors. It is a multiwave study that is still ongoing. The research, which is in part supported by the makers of Trojan condoms, has looked at the reported sexual behaviors of over 20,000 people in the United States ranging in age from 14 to 102 (National Survey of Sexual Health and Behavior, n.d.). According to the study, the reported rates of vaginal intercourse for men increases with age, at least for men in their 20s (National Survey of Sexual Health and Behavior, n.d.). For men ages 18–19, 52.8% reported having vaginal intercourse in the last year (Herbenick et al., 2010). This number increases to 85.7% for men ages 25–29 (Herbenick et al., 2010). Men reported being less likely to have been the recipient of anal sex than women, with 8.9% of men aged 18–24 reporting that they had engaged in this behavior in the last year, compared to 17% of women (Herbenick et al., 2010).

An analysis of oral sex behavior indicates men receive oral sex from their partner more often than they perform it. For men ages 18–24, 49.5% reported performing oral sex, compared to 57.3% of women, and 61.7% reported receiving oral sex in the last year, compared to 59.7% of women (Herbenick et al., 2010).

Regardless of which behaviors a person may choose to engage in, it's important that your partner gives consent to engage in those behaviors with you. Giving consent means that your partner willingly agrees to engage in a behavior and understands what that means. While it varies by location, in many countries, consent can't be given if a person is intoxicated or under the influence of drugs. It's also important to take steps to help limit the risk of contracting, or passing on, sexually transmitted infections (STIs). STIs will be discussed later in the chapter.

Consider this

While there is no one definition of sex, it's important that you understand how you define it, since it may impact what steps you take to protect against STIs and pregnancy.

Masturbation

Many people think of sex as being linked only to reproduction, but for many other people around the world the purpose of engaging in sex, or other sexual behaviors, might instead be pleasure. This is often the reason why people masturbate. Because statistics about masturbation are typically based on self-report, it is difficult to always get accurate rates. Some people, whether due to societal taboos, cultural and religious upbringing, or a sense of shame around sexual activity, may deny masturbating. In one study, 36% of German men, 41% of American men, and 48% of French men admitted to having lied about masturbating (Tenga, 2019). Tenga (2019) found that masturbation happens around the world, with the United Kingdom and Spain reporting the highest percentages of people masturbating, 91% and 93%, respectively. While the rates were lower in Korea (76%), Japan (76%), and China (73%), more than half of the people in those countries reported ever masturbating (Tenga, 2019).

While many believe that masturbation is a substitute for sex with a partner, that is not necessarily true. Recent research has shown that American men of all ages reported higher rates of solo masturbation than women (Regnerus, Price, & Gordon, 2017). Solo masturbation is masturbating by yourself, as opposed to masturbating with a partner present. The rates ranged from a low of 46% of men ages 70 and older to a high of 84% for men between the ages of 25–29 (Regnerus et al., 2017). Regnerus et al. (2017) did not identify a large difference in rates of masturbation between men ages 18–19 (81%) and 20–24 (83%). When researchers compared the rate of masturbation with a partner, the rates for men were higher than for women for all age groups, with the exception of 14–15 and 16–17 year olds (Regnerus et al., 2017).

Whether masturbation is often used to satisfy one's sexual needs, either with or without a partner, there are many other reasons why people may choose to masturbate. Masturbating allows a person to get to know their body and identify what feels good. They can then communicate this with their partners, making sexual activity more pleasurable. Some people find that masturbation helps them feel more energized, while others report that it helps them relax and fall asleep. There is some research that indicates that ejaculating multiple times a week may help reduce one's risk of prostate cancer, but the research on this is varied and ejaculation is not necessarily limited to masturbation (Aboul-Enein, Bernstein, & Ross, 2016). Ejaculation may be a result of a wet dream or partnered sexual behavior.

For many people, their views on masturbation are closely tied to what they learned about the behavior while growing up. While it is common in the United States to believe that men masturbate more than women, and this is supported by many surveys, it is also common for men to learn that it is sometimes considered deviant, since it's usually relegated to solo behavior or because it is viewed as being as acceptable as intercourse (Kaestle & Allen, 2011). Despite the fact that this can be considered to be safer sexual activity, since there is no risk of pregnancy, it is still a behavior that many report makes them feel ashamed or stigmatized (Kaestle & Allen, 2011).

In his own words

Anonymous, 33

I can remember a time talking to my dad on the phone, I was maybe 12 or so, that something was wrong with my eye, because it was very blurry. He told me that it was because I was masturbating; my parents had just caught me one morning. For the record, I scratched my cornea in gym class.

Learn more

Check out the Tenga Self-Pleasure report website www.feelmore.global/ to get more information on masturbation rates in Spain, Germany, France, the United Kingdom, and the United States.

Pornography

The consumption of pornography is not a new phenomenon linked to the internet. Before xtube and pornhub made porn free to anyone who could get to the website, porn was available on DVD, and before that on VCR tapes. Before people were sexting with their smartphones, they were sharing polaroid pictures of themselves. The *Merriam Webster Dictionary* (Pornography, n.d., para. 1) defines pornography as "the depiction of erotic behavior (as in pictures or writing) intended to cause sexual excitement." Using this definition, we can trace pornographic images back thousands of years to paintings done on cave walls.

Did you know?

What the internet has done is make pornography more accessible to people around the world. Information on popular pornography search terms in your country can be found at www.pornmd.com/sex-search.

With the ease of access to pornography today, and the almost complete lack of formal education on it, the concern for many is the impact that watching pornography can have on a person. Common concerns are that viewing pornography can lead to an increase in sexual violence, an increase in sexually risky behavior, a decrease in satisfaction with one-self and one's partner, and "porn addiction."

It's important to note that a lot of research involving pornography is inconclusive, often because the studies are biased and are designed to focus on the negative impact of pornography. This is especially true when looking at a possible association between viewing pornography and sexual violence. As noted by Ferguson and Hartley "evidence for a causal relationship between exposure to pornography and sexual aggression is slim and may, at certain times, have been exaggerated by politicians, pressure groups and some social scientists" (2009, p. 323).

Some of the research on pornography can be viewed positively. Recent research on college students in Germany and Poland found no association between watching pornography and having a high number of sexual partners (Martyniuk, Briken, Sehner, Richter-Appelt, & Dekker, 2016). In 2017, a meta-analysis was published that examined 50 studies from ten countries and found that there was no negative impact on how men who viewed pornography viewed themselves (Wright, Tokunga, Kraus, & Klann, 2017). However, that same meta-analysis did demonstrate an association between watching pornography and a decrease in satisfaction with one's partner, either in terms of satisfaction with their sex lives, or with relationship satisfaction (Wright et al., 2017).

For some people, there may be fear that they, or a loved one, has a "porn addiction." It's important to note that like sex addiction, porn addiction is not an actual disorder. They both lack any diagnostic criteria, which prevents an actual diagnosis of addiction. While some people may exhibit obsessive behaviors that center on pornography, for many, the issue of "porn addiction" is really a concern about the negative impact that viewing porn may have on them. It may have led to fights in a relationship about the amount of time that pornography is being watched, the partner feeling threatened, or having a reduction in satisfaction with one's partner.

Personal assessment

Most people ask if porn is good or bad, and there is no easy answer to that question. Much of the research evidence in this area is inconclusive. What it comes down to is how you feel about pornography. If watching it makes you feel guilty, if it goes against your morals and values, then perhaps it's not the right thing for you. Does watching it with your partner make your relationship stronger, or make you feel more comfortable with yourself? Then maybe it is good for you.

Kegel exercises

Discussion of men's sexual health in the media is limited in that the focus is often on the use of porn and its possible impact on relationships or transmission of STIs. What's often lacking is a discussion of what men can do to improve their sexual health, specifically the fact that Kegel exercises can be beneficial for men. Kegel exercises are named after gynecologist Dr. Arnold Kegel. For many women, incontinence (loss of bladder control) after childbirth is common, and Dr. Kegel introduced these exercises as a non-surgical way for women to address this issue. These exercises, which are now commonly referred to as pelvic floor exercises, involve repeatedly contracting and relaxing the pelvic floor muscles. These muscles, also known as the pubococcygeal muscles (PC) muscles, are present in all people, regardless of their sex. For men, doing Kegel exercises is as simple as tightening the PC muscles for 3–5 seconds, and then relaxing for 3–5 seconds. Men can do ten repetitions of this three times a day (MedlinePlus, 2019). For many men, the challenge is knowing which muscles they should be focusing on. One of the common suggestions for identifying these muscles is to start urinating and then stopping midstream. The muscles that allow you to stop urinating are the ones to focus on during the exercises. Remember to continue urinating once these muscles have been found.

There are a number of benefits, both sexual and nonsexual, for men who do Kegel exercises regularly. Doing these exercises regularly can help men who are struggling with incontinence, which may be caused by a number of factors, including having either an enlarged prostate or as a side effect of having a prostate removed. Alcohol and some prescription and non-prescription drugs can also cause incontinence in men (Bagnola, Pearce, & Broome, 2017).

Sexually, pelvic floor exercises can also be used to help men who have erectile dysfunction. A small pilot study involving ten men found that pelvic floor exercises in Indian men, along with lifestyle changes, led to a decrease in erectile dysfunction and an increase in sexual quality of life (Kumar & Sharif, 2017). Doing pelvic floor exercises may also be beneficial in that they can help men reach orgasm and can be a useful tool in helping men who have premature ejaculation (Cohen, Gonzalez, & Goldstein, 2016; Pasture et al., 2014). These exercises are less costly than other interventions and have no side effects like those seen from the use of SSRIs (Pasture et al., 2014). SSRIs are a type of antidepressant. For men who do not have a sexual dysfunction, there are still benefits to doing pelvic floor exercises. Strengthening the PC muscles can also lead to stronger orgasms.

Did you know?

WebMD provides information and specific how-to instructions for Kegel exercises in men (2018). To learn more, visit www.webmd.com/urinary-incontinence-oab/kegel-exercises-treating-male-urinary-incontinence#1.

STIs and STDs

STIs are infections that are transmitted through sexual activity, including oral, anal, and vaginal intercourse. STIs may be caused by many things, including viruses, bacteria, fungus, and protozoa. Many people have heard these referred to as sexually transmitted diseases (STDs) and although the two terms are often used interchangeably, they are not the same. A person has an STI when they have contracted an infection, but it is possible for that infection not to develop into a disease. As an example, someone may have been exposed to, and contracted the human papilloma virus (HPV). This means the person has an STI, but if they never show symptoms, or progress to a disease state, then technically, they do not have an STD. It is important to note the difference in terminology for several reasons. One is that there is a stigma that surrounds STDs and STIs. That stigma may prevent people from choosing to have discussion with their partners about any symptoms they may be experiencing and may cause them to delay going to a medical practitioner for a diagnosis. The treatment options may be different for someone who has an infection as compared to someone who is in a disease state.

With all STIs it's important to keep in mind that a person who has been diagnosed can still have an active sex life. If someone has been diagnosed, it's important for them to be open with their partners about their diagnosis and discuss steps that they can take to help reduce the chances of spreading the infection. This may include not engaging in contact with the genitals during a herpes outbreak or abstaining from vaginal, anal, and oral sex until treatment is complete for a bacterial infection, such as chlamydia.

There are many common STIs that impact men. The rates of the two most common bacterial STIs, which are gonorrhea and chlamydia, have been increasing in men. Gonorrhea rates have been steadily increasing in the United States since 2009, and since 2013 there has been a greater increase in rates among males than females. In 2016, the rates of gonorrhea rose from 139.7 per 100,000 males to 170.7, which is an increase of 22.2% (Centers for Disease Control and Prevention (CDC), 2017b). This is greater than the 13.8% increase among women (CDC, 2017b). Among men in the United States, gonorrhea rates were highest among those aged 20–24. There are some regional differences in gonorrhea rates, as the highest rates were reported in the South in 2016 (CDC, 2017b). These numbers are high when compared to the rest of the world. In 2016, the median global rate of gonorrhea in men in 64 countries was 18.8 per 100,000 (World Health Organization (WHO), 2018).

Similar to gonorrhea, there has been an increase in the reported cases of chlamydia over the last few years. While there are more reported cases of chlamydia in women, there has been a larger increase in the rates among men since 2012. Currently, women's rates of chlamydia are significantly higher than men's. In 2016, there were a reported 657.3 cases per 100,000 in women compared to 330.5 per 100,000 in men (CDC, 2017c). From 2012 to 2016, there was a 26.5% increase of chlamydia rates in men compared to a 2.9% increase among women in that same timeframe (CDC, 2017c).

The most common symptoms of both gonorrhea and chlamydia in men are a burning sensation when urinating and a discharge from the penis (CDC, 2014). This discharge may be yellow, white or green (Planned Parenthood, n.d.). It is important to note that there are some men who may not experience any symptoms, despite being infected. If a man was the receptive partner during anal intercourse, he may experience bleeding or discharge from the anus or anal itching with gonorrhea.

Testing for gonorrhea can be done using a urine test. This test can be done at home, though often it is done at a doctor's office or clinic. If there are concerns about gonorrhea in the anus or throat, then a swab in those areas will need to be used. It may take 2–3 days for the results from the test to become available. If infected, the most common treatment is a combination of two antibiotics, however, over the last decade there has been evidence of an increase in the cases of antibiotic-resistant gonorrhea worldwide (Deresinski, 2017).

Treatment for chlamydia may be one of several antibiotics. A medical practitioner will decide which is best. Regardless of which antibiotic is prescribed, it's important that people take all their medication and that they do not have unprotected intercourse while they are being treated. If a person has regular sexual partners, they should also be tested so that the bacteria is not continuously spread back and forth.

Syphilis is another STI that is caused by bacteria. Syphilis, if left untreated, will progress through multiple stages. Primary stage syphilis is usually indicated by a sore that can be found where the body came into contact with the virus. For example, if someone had unprotected penile-vaginal intercourse and was exposed to syphilis, the sore would appear on the penis. If left untreated, the sore will go away, but the infection is not gone. At this point, the person will develop secondary syphilis, which usually presents as a rash and fever (CDC, 2017c). Eventually, the symptoms of secondary syphilis will disappear and the person will enter the latent stage. During this stage, the person will show no symptoms. The latent stage can last for years. The last stage of syphilis is the tertiary stage, and it is the most severe, often marked by organ damage. A blood test is used to determine if a person has syphilis. The blood can be taken from a vein, or a simple finger stick. Treatment for syphilis is antibiotics.

While once on the decline, the rates of syphilis in the United States have been increasing since 2001 (CDC, 2018). From 2016 to 2017, 72% of states and Washington DC, saw an increase in the rates of primary and secondary syphilis (CDC, 2018). This increase is not seen worldwide. A meta-analysis indicates that there has been a general decrease in syphilis worldwide over the past 30 years, although the rates are higher in sub-Saharan Africa (Smolak et al., 2018).

In addition to bacterial STIs, there are three common STIs that are caused by viruses. These include herpes, HIV, and HPV. There are over 100 different strains of HPV, but not all of them can be spread sexually. Some of these strains cause warts, while others may cause certain types of cancer, including penile and anal cancer. If a person is exposed to HPV in their throat, it can lead to cancer at the back of the throat. These types of cancer are rare.

HPV is incredibly common in the United States and most people's bodies can clear it within two years of exposure. It's hard to get accurate numbers of HPV infection rates in the United States, as it is not one of the infections that are required to be reported to the CDC. Genital warts are caused by HPV, and recent estimates indicate that one in every 100 sexually active adults have genital warts at any given time (CDC, 2019a). But this estimate may be low since not everyone who has a wart seeks treatment from a health care provider.

There are several vaccines available to help prevent the spread of HPV. These vaccines are available worldwide. In the United States, the current recommendation is for boys and men between the ages of 11 and 45 to be vaccinated (CDC, 2019b). In many countries, the targets for vaccines are females, so males may not be utilizing the vaccine. HPV is spread through skin-to-skin contact, so condoms are not 100% effective at preventing transmission. There are no screenings for HPV for men, but if you notice something that looks like a wart in the genital or anal area it's important to get it checked out. It's important to keep in mind that the strains of HPV that cause warts don't cause cancer. However, it is possible to have multiple strains of HPV at the same time, and throughout one's lifetime.

For men, there are no routine tests for genital warts. If a doctor sees something that they suspect is a wart, they can put a vinegar solution on it to see if it changes color (WebMD, 2017). It's important to note that this is not a perfect test. For men who engage in receptive anal sex, a pap test can be done. This involves collecting anal cells and examining them for signs of abnormalities (WebMD, 2017).

Genital warts can be removed but, depending on size and location, they may just be allowed to go away on their own. Removal can be through a variety of methods, including topical medications, cryotherapy, or surgery.

Another virus-caused STI is herpes simplex virus, or HSV. HSV is typically referred to as herpes. There are many different viruses in the herpes family. Epstein-Barr virus, and the virus that causes mononucleosis, are in the herpes family, as is chicken pox (varicella zoster virus). When most people talk about herpes and sex, they are referring to HSV-1 or HSV-2.

In previous decades, there used to be a distinction made between HSV-1 and HSV-2. HSV-1 was commonly referred to as "oral herpes" because it causes cold sores on and around the lips, and HSV-2 was commonly associated with genital herpes. Because HSV-1 can cause genital infections through oral sex (the person infected with HSV on their mouth performs oral sex on someone), many medical practices do not make a distinction between the two viruses.

HSV is a common virus in the United States. The estimates are that more than one out of six people between the ages of 14 and 49 have it (CDC, 2017a). HSV is also common around the world. According to WHO, 67% of people under the age of 50 have HSV-1 (2015). In every region of the world, with the exception of the Americas and Europe, the prevalence of HSV-1 is higher for men than women (WHO, 2015).

If a person has HSV it does not necessarily mean that they have outbreaks. Most people who have genital herpes will either show no symptoms, or symptoms that are mild. These symptoms include small blisters or sores. When there are symptoms, they usually appear as a sore or two. It is possible to spread herpes even if there are no symptoms. Herpes can be spread by skin-to-skin contact, contact with saliva if someone has oral herpes, or contact with genital secretions. A herpes diagnosis may be visual, in that a medical professional determines that a sore or blister is herpes by examining it. Additionally, a blood test can be done.

Being diagnosed with herpes, or any other STI, does not mean that you can't have a healthy sex life. You should be honest with your partners about your diagnosis and discuss ways to help reduce the risk of spreading it to them. One way to prevent spreading the virus is to make sure to use a barrier method, such as an external (male) or internal (female) condom, every time you have oral, anal, or vaginal intercourse. If you have been diagnosed with herpes, your doctor might prescribe an antiviral medication to reduce the intensity and duration of the current outbreak. If you have recurrent outbreaks, your doctor may prescribe a daily medication to reduce the likelihood of future outbreaks.

Human immunodeficiency virus (simply known as HIV) is the virus that causes acquired immune deficiency syndrome (AIDS). How a diagnosis of HIV is managed has changed substantially over the last few decades. In the 1980s, a person diagnosed with HIV quickly moved to an AIDS diagnosis and then died. Today, an HIV diagnosis is looked at more as a long-term chronic disease that can be managed with medication. The sooner someone is diagnosed, the sooner they can begin treatment.

Should you get tested?

The sooner a person finds out they're HIV positive, the sooner they can begin treatment, so early diagnosis is important. And since many places offer free HIV testing, maybe you should ask yourself why shouldn't you get tested?

Websites to help you find HIV testing sites:
In Europe: www.ecdc.europa.eu/en/test-finder
In Canada: www.cdnaids.ca/resources/hiv-information-hotlines/
In the United States: https://gettested.cdc.gov/

HIV can be passed through contact with semen, blood, breast milk, and vaginal secretions. It cannot be passed through casual contact, like hugging, or through saliva. An HIV diagnosis is made if someone tests positive on an HIV test. The HIV test may be done using a blood or oral fluid sample. With rapid testing, results can be determined in 20 minutes. It is important to note that if someone thinks they have been exposed to HIV, they should wait at least three weeks before getting tested. These three weeks, which is referred to as a window period, is a time when the body is making antibodies to the virus, and many HIV tests are designed to detect these antibodies.

If someone is diagnosed with HIV it's important to connect with a health care provider who can help determine next steps. There are many medications that are available that can reduce their viral load and slow the progression to later stage HIV (often referred to as AIDS). An AIDS diagnosis is made after a person has tested positive for HIV and either has a T cell count below 200 per cubic millimeter, or has one or more diseases that are often referred to as opportunistic infections.

The viral load is the amount of virus in a person's bloodstream, and thanks to newer medications and treatment regimens, the viral load for some people has gotten so low it is undetectable. In these situations, this means that the person can no longer transmit HIV. For this to happen, a person with HIV needs to know that they have the virus and begin taking medications. This is another reason why it's important to get tested.

Another reason to get tested is that if someone has HIV they can tell their partner, and they can take steps to protect themselves from contracting the disease. For people who engage in sexual activity with people who have HIV, there is a daily pill they can take which can help reduce their risk of contracting HIV. This option, called PrEP (pre-exposure prophylaxis) has been shown to decrease a person's chances of acquiring HIV (Fonner et al., 2016).

Did you know?

Not sure if you're at risk for HIV? Check out this website http://checkhimout.ca/testing/know-your-risk/know-your-risk/.

Impact of BPA on male fertility

For some men, having an untreated STI can lead to future infertility (Ochsendorf, 2008). Over the years, there has been much debate about what other factors may impact a man's fertility. Infertility for men is when a man cannot get a woman pregnant after a year of trying (U.S. Department of Health and Human Services, 2019). The estimates are that one-third of all infertility cases are caused by male infertility (U.S. National Library of Medicine, 2018). There are many potential causes of male infertility, ranging from hormonal imbalances, to scarring from STIs, to a decrease in sperm count due to aging (Olooto, 2017). In addition to these causes, doctors also look at lifestyle factors to determine their potential impact on sperm development and hormonal imbalances. These lifestyle factors may include smoking tobacco and drinking alcohol (Kumar, Murarka, Mishra, & Gautam, 2014). There has been some discussion in the media about the role of everything from bike shorts to laptop computers on male infertility (Alvero, 2013; Fertility Centers of Illinois, n.d.). A recent possible link to male infertility has focused on xenoestrogen bisphenol-A (BPA). BPA is a chemical that can be found in many products from water bottles, to CDs, to the lining of canned foods. Many manufacturers of items that have used BPA in the past have now switched to other chemicals, and are creating BPA-free products. Over the last decade, there have been individual studies that have found a potential link between BPA exposure and male infertility. But a review of the available studies indicates that there are no consistent findings to suggest this link (Mínguez-Alarcón, Hauser, & Gaskins, 2016).

This is an emerging area in research in male infertility. If a man is concerned about his fertility, instead of focusing solely on BPA he may want to be aware of other lifestyle factors and seek medical advice from a trusted health professional.

Did you know?

The Environmental Working Group recommends the documentary *The Disappearing Male* to anyone wishing to learn more about the impact of hormone disruptors (2008). The documentary is available online on various websites.

Moving forward

Safe sex campaigns that target men, often focus on men who have sex with men, such as the social media campaign that ran on Facebook and apps like Grindr that was launched in Canada after there was an outbreak of syphilis (Ross et al., 2016). While it's important to target those at highest risk, those who do not identify as a man who has sex with men may not be impacted by the campaign.

A recent campaign in Alaska, called "Wrap it up Alaska" (iknowmine.org, n. d.), targeted teens to try to prevent chlamydia (Figure 5.1). One of the ways that safe sex education has been increasing on college campuses is through Sex Weeks. While these types of campus events are informative and often well attended, there have been concerns on the part of some campus administrators that are limiting these types of events (Mulhere, 2014).

Many people equate sexual health with women's health, since women are statistically more likely to contract an STI when having sex with men, and since women are the ones who can get pregnant. This needs to change. We need to involve men more in these conversations about condoms, STIs, and contraception, not just for their partner's health, but also for their own. We need to provide men with information on sexual health and create spaces where they feel comfortable going for care.

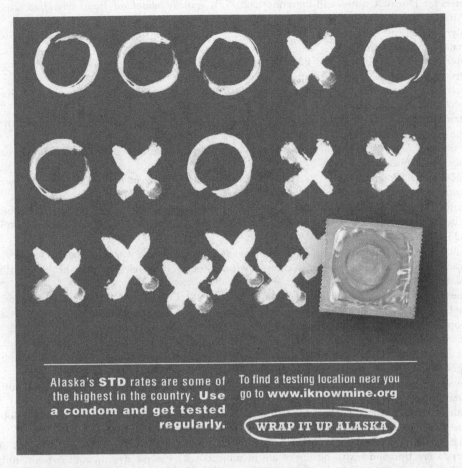

Figure 5.1 Hugs and kisses poster. This advertisement from Wrap it up Alaska promotes condoms, regular STD testing, and where to find testing locations.

Source: Developed by iknowmine.org.

References

Aboul-Enein, B. H., Bernstein, J., & Ross, M. W. (2016). Evidence for masturbation and prostate cancer risk: Do we have a verdict? *Sexual Medicine Reviews, 4*(3), 229–234.

Alvero, R. (2013). How bicycling affects male fertility. *Advanced Reproductive Medicine. University of Colorado.* Retrieved from https://arm.coloradowomenshealth.com/doctors-blog/bicycling-affect-male-fertility

Bagnola, E., Pearce, E., & Broome, B. (2017). A review and case study of urinary incontinence. *Madridge Journal of Nursing, 2*(1), 27–31.

Centers for Disease Control and Prevention. (2014). *Gonorrhea – CDC fact sheet.* Retrieved from www.cdc.gov/std/gonorrhea/stdfact-gonorrhea.htm

Centers for Disease Control and Prevention. (2017a). *Genital herpes – CDC fact sheet.* Retrieved from www.cdc.gov/std/herpes/stdfact-herpes.htm

Centers for Disease Control and Prevention. (2017b). *Syphilis – CDC fact sheet.* Retrieved from www.cdc.gov/std/syphilis/stdfact-syphilis.htm

Centers for Disease Control and Prevention. (2017c). *Sexually transmitted disease surveillance 2016*. Atlanta: U.S. Department of Health and Human Services.

Centers for Disease Control and Prevention. (2018). *Syphilis*. Retrieved from www.cdc.gov/std/stats17/syphilis.htm

Centers for Disease Control and Prevention. (2019a). *HPV and men – fact sheet*. Retrieved from www.cdc.gov/std/hpv/stdfact-hpv-and-men.htm

Centers for Disease Control and Prevention. (2019b). *Vaccinating boys and girls*. Retrieved from www.cdc.gov/hpv/parents/vaccine.html

Cohen, D., Gonzalez, J., & Goldstein, I. (2016). The role of pelvic floor muscles in male sexual dysfunction and pelvic pain. *Sexual Medicine Reviews, 4*(1), 53–62.

Deresinski, S. (2017). GASP! Increasing worldwide antibiotic resistance in neisseria gonorrhoeae. *Infectious Disease Alert, 36*(11).

Environmental Working Group. (2008). *The Disappearing Male documents concerning issues*. Retrieved from www.ewg.org/enviroblog/2008/11/disappearing-male-documents-concerning-issues

Ferguson, C. J., & Hartley, R. D. (2009). The pleasure is momentary … the expense damnable? The influence of pornography on rape and sexual assault. *Aggression and Violent Behavior, 14*(5), 323–329.

Fertility Centers of Illinois. (n.d.). *Men's health month: 11 male infertility myths debunked*. Retrieved from https://fcionline.com/our-center/news-and-media/press-releases/mens-health-month-11-male-infertility-myths-debunked/

Fonner, V. A., Dalglish, S. L., Kennedy, C. E., Baggaley, R., O'Reilly, K. R., Koechlin, F. M., … & Grant, R. M. (2016). Effectiveness and safety of oral HIV preexposure prophylaxis for all populations. *AIDS (London, England), 30*(12), 1973.

Herbenick, D., Reece, M., Schick, V., Sanders, S. A., Dodge, B., & Fortenberry, J. D. (2010). Sexual behavior in the United States: Results from a national probability sample of men and women ages 14–94. *The Journal of Sexual Medicine, 7*, 255–265.

Iknowmine.org. (n.d.). *Wrap it up Alaska*. Retrieved from www.iknowmine.org/other-cool-stuff/wrapitupak

Kaestle, C. E., & Allen, K. R. (2011). The role of masturbation in healthy sexual development: Perceptions of young adults. *Archives of Sexual Behavior, 40*(5), 983–994.

Kumar, G. N. J., & Sharif, S. I. (2017). Effects of pelvic floor muscle strengthening exercises on penile erection and sexual quality of life in subjects with erectile dysfunction: A pilot study. *Indian Journal of Physiotherapy and Rehabilitation, 1*(1), 27–31.

Kumar, S., Murarka, S., Mishra, V. V., & Gautam, A. K. (2014). Environmental & lifestyle factors in deterioration of male reproductive health. *The Indian Journal of Medical Research, 140*(Suppl 1), S29–S35.

Martyniuk, U., Briken, P., Sehner, S., Richter-Appelt, H., & Dekker, A. (2016). Pornography use and sexual behavior among Polish and German university students. *Journal of Sex & Marital Therapy, 42*(6), 494–514.

MedlinePlus. (2019). *Kegel exercises: Self-care*. Retrieved from https://medlineplus.gov/ency/patientinstructions/000141.htm

Mínguez-Alarcón, L., Hauser, R., & Gaskins, A. J. (2016). Effects of bisphenol A on male and couple reproductive health: A review. *Fertility and Sterility, 106*(4), 864–870.

Mulhere, K. (2014). *Red-faced over sex weeks*. Retrieved from www.insidehighered.com/news/2014/10/15/sex-week-events-draw-criticism-some-campuses

National Survey of Sexual Health and Behavior. (n.d.). Retrieved from www.nationalsexstudy.indiana.edu/

Ochsendorf, F. R. (2008). Sexually transmitted infections: Impact on male fertility. *Andrologia, 40*(2), 72–75.

Olooto, W. E. (2017). Infertility in male; risk factors, causes and management: A review. *Journal of Microbiology and Biotechnology Research, 2*(4), 641–645.

Pasture, A. L., Palleschi, G., Fuschi, A., Maggioni, C., Rago, R., Zucchi, A., & Carbone, A. (2014). Pelvic floor muscle rehabilitation for patients with lifelong premature ejaculation: A novel therapeutic approach. *Therapeutic Advances in Urology*, *6*(3), 83–88.

Planned Parenthood. (n.d.). *What are the symptoms of gonorrhea?* Retrieved from www.plannedparenthood.org/learn/stds-hiv-safer-sex/gonorrhea/what-are-symptoms-gonorrhea

Pornography. (n.d.). *In Merriam Webster.* Retrieved from www.merriam-webster.com/dictionary/pornography

Regnerus, M., Price, J., & Gordon, D. (2017). Masturbation and partnered sex: Substitutes or complements? *Archives of Sexual Behavior*, *46*(7), 2111–2121.

Ross, C., Shaw, S., Marshall, S., Stephen, S., Bailey, K., Cole, R., … & Plourde, P. (2016). Update on STIs: Impact of a social media campaign targeting men who have sex with men during an outbreak of syphilis in Winnipeg, Canada. *Canada Communicable Disease Report*, *42*(2), 45.

Smolak, A., Rowley, J., Nagelkerke, N., Kassebaum, N. J., Chico, R. M., Korenromp, E. L., & Abu-Raddad, L. J. (2018). Trends and predictors of syphilis prevalence in the general population: Global pooled analyses of 1103 prevalence measures including 136 million syphilis tests. *Clinical Infectious Diseases*, *66*(8), 1184–1191.

Tenga. (2019). *2019 Self-pleasure report.* Retrieved from www.feelmore.global/wp-content/uploads/2019/05/TENGA-BCW-2019-Global-Survey-US-Report-5.10.19.pdf

U.S. Department of Health and Human Services. (2019). *Male infertility.* Retrieved from www.hhs.gov/opa/reproductive-health/fact-sheets/male-infertility/index.html

U.S. National Library of Medicine. (2018). *Male infertility.* Retrieved from https://medlineplus.gov/maleinfertility.html

WebMD. (2017). *HPV infections in men.* Retrieved from www.webmd.com/sexual-conditions/hpv-genital-warts/hpv-virus-men#1

World Health Organization. (2015). *Globally, an estimated two-thirds of the population under 50 are infected with herpes simplex virus type 1.* Retrieved from www.who.int/news-room/detail/28-10-2015-globally-an-estimated-two-thirds-of-the-population-under-50-are-infected-with-herpes-simplex-virus-type-1

World Health Organization. (2018). *Report on global sexually transmitted infection surveillance 2018.*

Wright, P. J., Tokunaga, R. S., Kraus, A., & Klann, E. (2017). Pornography consumption and satisfaction: A meta-analysis. *Human Communication Research*, *43*(3), 315–343.

6 Sexual orientation

Diana Karczmarczyk and Courtney M. Gonzalez

Definitions

There is much confusion about the difference between sex and gender identity and how these relate to sexual orientation. This chapter will provide a brief overview of each of these terms. Sex and gender are often used interchangeably, and this is confusing because these two terms have key distinctions. Sex is typically separated into the two biological categories of male and female based on reproductive functions. For example, male species provide sperm and female species provide eggs. A person's sex is typically assigned at birth based on external anatomy. Although this type of sex assignment is common practice, just under 2% of individuals are born with external anatomy, internal anatomy, or chromosomes that may not align within the binary system, commonly referred to as intersex people (interACT, n.d.). The binary system refers to the rigid belief that individuals fall into one of two options such as either male or female. New York City was the first jurisdiction in the United States to pass legislation for a third option on birth certificates to include intersex in 2016, followed by the state of Colorado in 2018 (Sakas, 2018). The United Nations (n.d.) reports that Australia, in 2013, was the first nation to pass legislation protecting intersex people from discrimination, followed by Malta in 2015.

Learn more

At eight months of age, Bruce Reimer, who was born in Canada in 1965, had his penis burned off when a circumcision went awry (Colapinto, 2000). In the book *As Nature Made Him: The boy who was raised as a girl* by John Colapinto, you can learn more about the recommended sex reassignment that was recommended by experts at the time and the impact of this on the whole family.

Unlike sex, gender identity is not based on biology, but rather on social constructs. Social constructs are expectations and values that society places on an individual's behavior (World Health Organization (WHO), 2019). For example, society may expect that the role of a man includes providing financial security and stability to their family unit. Cisgender is the term used when a person's assigned sex at birth aligns with these social constructs. Gender expectations can be understood and exhibited differently across the globe. Gender identity is often described as how people view themselves. Individuals that view themselves in contradiction to rigid social constructs experience health disparities and discrimination, which are discussed in this chapter.

In the acronym LGBTQ, the letters LGB stand for lesbian, gay, and bisexual and refer to sexual orientation. Sexual orientation is used to describe the complex interplay of emotional, physical, and sexual attraction a person may feel (Gender Spectrum, 2019). The letter T in the LGBTQ acronym refers to transgender, which refers to a person's gender identity. Gender Spectrum explains that transgender is used "to describe anyone whose gender identity differs from their assigned sex" (2019, para. 22). Since transgender is included in this commonly used acronym, it may be confusing since a person's gender identity does not imply their sexual orientation. The letter Q in the LGBTQ acronym can refer to people who are questioning either their gender identity or their sexual orientation. The letter Q may also be used by people who identify as queer (Grinberg, 2019). PFLAG explains that queer is a term that mostly young people use when they do not self-identify with a binary system that extends beyond male and female or straight and gay (2019).

The term sexual and gender minority, or SGM, is often used in research when referring to LGBTQ individuals as an umbrella term, particularly when addressing their unique health concerns and the disparities in health outcomes. This term will be used throughout the chapter.

The Kinsey Scale, also known as the Heterosexual-Homosexual Rating Scale, was developed by the prominent sex researcher Alfred Kinsey in 1948 (Kinsey Institute, 2018). Kinsey used this 7-point scale in his research to describe sexual orientation, which he believed to be fluid. On one end of the scale (0) were individuals whose sexual desires and/or experiences were exclusively heterosexual, while on the other end were those whose sexual desires and/or experiences were exclusively homosexual (6); in-between (1–5) were individuals with varying levels of desire for and/or experiences with both sexes (Kinsey Institute, 2018). Kinsey's scale demonstrated that people did not fit neatly into exclusive heterosexual or homosexual categories. However, it did not actually reference how individuals identified or labeled their own sexual identity.

The Klein Sexual Orientation Grid, also referred to as KSOG, was developed by sex researcher Dr. Fritz Klein in 1978 on the premise that sexual orientation is an "ongoing dynamic process" (American Institute of Bisexuality [AIB], 2014b, para. 4) and "too complex to be broken into simple, well-defined categories" (AIB, 2014a, para. 5). AIB (2014b) shares that Dr. Klein first introduced this tool in his book *The Bisexual Option* outlining seven components of sexual orientation.

Personal assessment

Visit https://bi.org/en/klein-grid to complete the KSOG and learn about the various components of your own sexual orientation.

When referring to sexual orientation, it is important to use appropriate and respectful language. GLAAD explains that the term gay can be used to identify "people whose enduring physical, romantic, and/or emotional attractions are to people of the same sex"; therefore, the phrases gay man or gay people are acceptable phrases to use (n.d., para. 2). However, it is not acceptable to use the term homosexual because this is an "outdated term considered derogatory and offensive to many lesbian and gay people" (GLAAD, n.d., para. 2). It is also important to note that a person's sexual behavior does not define their sexual orientation either. A man may have sex with another man, referred to as MSM, and not identify as gay, emphasizing that sexual behavior does not equate with sexual orientation.

Statistics

According to a 2018 Gallup poll, the number of Americans who identify as LGBT increased to 4.5% in 2018 up from 3.5% in 2012 (Newport, 2018). Among the estimated 11.5 million individuals that identify as LGBT, females continue to be more likely to identify as LGBT than males (Newport, 2018). Since 2012, the number of females who self-identified as LGBT rose from 3.5% to 5.1%, while the number of males who self-identified as LGBT rose slightly from 3.4% to 3.9% (Newport, 2018). The data for the number of Americans that identify as LBGT remains consistent among sources.

Did you know?

Human Rights Watch tracks policies and publishes reports on the global rights of lesbian, gay, bisexual, transgender, and intersex (LGBTI) people (2019). Learn more at www.hrw.org/topic/lgbt-rights.

It is difficult to determine the total number of LGBT people across the globe. International data indicates between 1.5% and 7.4% of adults identify as LGBT (Deveaux, 2016). The Williams Institute conducts research on sexual orientation and in 2011 released a research brief exploring the challenges in data collection and population estimates of LGBT people around the world (Gates, 2011). The author explains that inconsistencies in language used in survey questions may result in data that may be difficult to analyze (Gates, 2011). Specifically, the concern is that "[i]dentity, behavior, attraction, and relationships all capture related dimensions of sexual orientation but none of these measures completely addresses the concept" (Gates, 2011, p. 2). For example, Gates (2011) recommends that survey tools also examine gender identity and the comparison to their sex assigned at birth. Deveaux (2016) also explains that answering questions about sexuality may be a sensitive topic and that using tools to protect respondent anonymity may result in more accurate data. The inconsistencies in the data are also evident in this chapter, as some of the information presented applies only to LGB individuals at times and LGBTQ at other times. Data may also be difficult to ascertain globally because there are laws in place that may discourage individuals from being out, a term used when a person discloses that they are LGBTQ, without jeopardizing their physical safety.

Learn more

Director Hao Wu's documentary, *All in My Family* (2019), is the story of a Chinese filmmaker who wants to come out to his traditional and socially conservative extended family (Global, 2019).

In his own words

Steven M.

After college I moved to DC, which was quite a change. Men would hold hands walking down the street and the level of acceptance was like no other; however, at the same time I really wanted to be part of the U.S. Foreign Service. Unfortunately, at that time, neither the United States nor the State Department recognized gay relationships. I knew that I could be sent to serve in a country where the consequences of being gay were a matter of life and death. Although I would have been covered by diplomatic immunity, not being able to live my life and, meet, and potentially date, men was disheartening, to say the least. So, I made the decision not to join the State Department. I often wondered about this decision and if that was the best approach for me being a young gay male.

Global policies

In June 2015, the U.S. Supreme Court upheld the rights for same-sex couples (5–4) to marry in the case of *Obergefell v. Hodges* and legalized same-sex marriage. By 2017, more than 10% of LGBT adults were married in the United States, with slightly more LGBT men (11.4%) than LGBT women (9.3%) reporting being married (Jones, 2017). Across the globe, over two dozen countries, mostly in Europe and the Americas, have also legalized same-sex marriage. These include, but are not limited to, Germany, Ireland, Brazil, France, Canada, and Iceland (Pew Research, 2019). In addition, South Africa and Taiwan joined these nations in legalizing same-sex marriage in 2006 and 2019, respectively (Pew Research, 2019).

Learn more

In the 2008 film, *Milk*, director Gus Van Sant unfolds the story of Harvey Milk, a gay rights activist and the first openly gay man elected to public office in California (Focus Features, 2019).

Every year, The International Lesbian, Gay, Bisexual, Trans and Intersex Association (ILGA) publishes a map of the world indicating the sexual orientation laws around the world (ILGA, n.d.; see Figure 6.1). The map distinguishes countries based on policies that either protect against discrimination based on sexual orientation or criminalize sex acts between consenting adults. Policies range from constitutional protections to the death penalty. For example, Bolivia has constitutional protections in place to protect individuals against discrimination based on sexual orientation, while Ukraine's protections are limited to discrimination based on sexual orientation in the workplace (ILGA, n.d.). In contrast, multiple countries in the Middle East criminalize sex acts between adults of the same sex, punishable with the death penalty (ILGA, n.d.). This reality can be dangerous for LGBT individuals. There are also several countries, such as India, China, and the Russian Federation, that do not have policies that either protect against discrimination

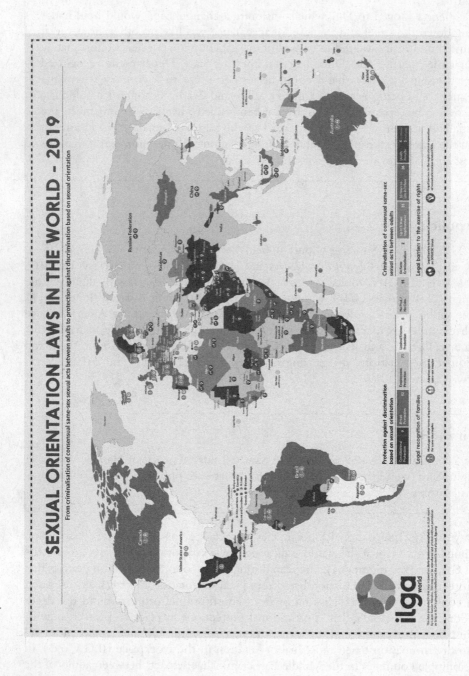

Figure 6.1 Map depicting sexual orientation laws in the world, 2019.

Source: Developed by The International Lesbian, Gay, Bisexual, Trans and Intersex Association. Retrieved from https://ilga.org/maps-sexual-orientation-laws.

or criminalize sex acts between same-sex adults, but have barriers in place to prevent individuals from expressing their sexual orientation, gender identity, or sex characteristics (ILGA, n.d.).

Furthermore, ILGA (2019) identifies countries with policies on same-sex marriage and adoption. Most countries that provide some level of legal protection against discrimination based on sexual orientation also legalize marriage or same-sex unions. Furthermore, these countries also legalized adoptions without restrictions based on sexual orientation. The Movement Advancement Project (MAP) tracks policies that protect LGBT families in the United States (MAP, 2019). For example, 41 states do not have laws that protect LGBT families against discrimination to foster youth and 42 states do not have laws to protect against discrimination in adoption based on sexual orientation or gender identity (MAP, 2019). Perrin, Hurley, Mattern, Flavin, and Pinderhughes (2019) found that more than 60% of 732 gay fathers across 47 states had experienced stigma at least once in the past year. For example, when a pediatrician refuses to assess a six-day-old baby because the parents are a same-sex couple which goes against the doctor's religious beliefs (Human Rights Watch, 2018). Despite the lack in legal protections and support, research supports that gay fathers are able to raise healthy children. An online survey of 61 gay fathers in two states highlighted that despite the stigma associated with being a same-sex couple raising a child, their children were just as healthy as their peers (Perrin, Pinderhughes, Mattern, Hurley, & Newman, 2016). Acknowledging that being a parent can be difficult, Erez and Shenkman (2016) compared survey data from 90 gay fathers and 90 heterosexual fathers in Israel and found that the subjective wellbeing of gay fathers was higher and their children thrived, indicating that their family structure was positive for the parents and child(ren).

Did you know?

Iceland proudly markets the legal protections provided for all people including marriage and adoptions on the marketing website for Visit Reykjavík. Visitors can learn about these protections and the vast number of "gay friendly travel destinations" and Pride events celebrated annually in August (visitreykjavik.is, 2019, para. 1).

Current research

To date, a leading question asked about sexual orientation is whether someone is born gay. This question has been the subject of multiple research efforts. In August 2019, the results of the largest sexuality research study were released. Ganna et al. (2019) reviewed DNA samples from over 480,000 participants and concluded that there is no single gene or a few genes responsible for sexual orientation, confirming that sexual orientation is complex and likely influenced by thousands of genes and the environment.

Did you know?

The largest LGBT health care, research, and education facility in the world is located in Boston, Massachusetts (Fenway Health, 2019). Learn more about Fenway Health at https://fenwayhealth.org/.

Health disparities

Similar to other minority groups, the LGBTQ community encounters a vast range of health disparities. It is also important to note that intersectionality can be present, compounding health disparities due to being a member of several minority populations, for example a black gay man. Some reasons to help explain why these disparities exist are lack of representation in research, little recognition of being a minority population, relatively small population size, and negative attitudes about SGM (Wolitski, Valdiserri, & Stall, 2007).

In 2017, 63% of all new HIV infections in adults occurred in men across the globe (UNAIDS, 2018). Of the most notable health disparities among MSM is the disproportionate rate of HIV. According to the Centers for Disease Control and Prevention (CDC) (2019b), gay and bisexual men made up 70% of new HIV diagnoses for 2017 within the United States. Although there is not a total estimate of the global impact of HIV specifically among MSM, it has been reported that globally MSM are 27 times more likely to acquire HIV (Avert, 2019b). More than half of all new HIV infections in North America, central Europe, and western Europe are among MSM (UNAIDS, 2018). When considering the intersectionality of race and sexual identity, black gay and bisexual men in the United States account for 37% of all new HIV diagnoses among the MSM population (CDC, 2019a). The high rates of HIV among MSM globally are associated with high rates of HIV-related cancers, such as anal cancer (Wolitski et al., 2007). MSM are also disproportionately affected by hepatitis B (Wolitski et al., 2007) and syphilis (CDC, 2017).

Did you know?

Individuals at risk for anal cancer are encouraged to discuss available screening tests. In the United States, although there is not an exam available to screen for anal cancer, a digital rectal exam, called a DRE, or an anal Pap test may be helpful in identifying anal cancer early (American Cancer Society, 2019).

Through cross-sectional surveys, it has been found that SGMs misuse substances at higher rates when compared to other populations (National Institute on Drug Abuse [NIDA], 2017). It has been thought to be associated with the discrimination and harassment that LGBTQ people constantly endure (NIDA, 2017). A study conducted by the U.S. Census Bureau reported higher rates of binge drinking in LGBT people than in heterosexual counterparts (Ward, Dahlhamer, Galinsky, & Joestl, 2014); additionally LGBT people have also reported earlier initiation of alcohol consumption (McCabe, West, Hughes, & Boyd, 2013). As for drug misuse, LGBTQ people have been found to have higher rates of misusing prescription pain relievers in addition to consuming more marijuana (NIDA, 2017). Substance use among this population has also been associated with their rates of HIV due to risky sexual behavior while under the influence (NIDA, 2017).

Substance use rates are also associated with issues of mental health among LGBTQ people. As discussed above, LGBTQ individuals endure excessive harassment and discrimination. With each negative encounter, it is estimated that the likelihood to self-harm increases 2.5 times (Mustanski, Garofalo, & Emerson, 2010). LGBTQ youth experience higher rates of suicidal ideation than LGBTQ adults (National Alliance on Mental

Illness [NAMI], 2019). However, LGB adults still experience higher rates of mental health conditions than heterosexual counterparts (NAMI, 2019). Transgender individuals experience tremendously high rates of suicidal ideation when compared with the general U.S. population (NAMI, 2019). In addition to suicidal ideations, LGBTQ individuals are at a higher risk of developing an eating disorder. Although gay men only make up a small percentage of the overall male population, it is estimated that 42% have an eating disorder (National Eating Disorders Association [NEDA], 2018). Factors that may influence the likelihood of developing an eating disorder are similar to those that cause LGBTQ individuals to endure negative mental health outcomes. Some factors include harassment, violence, discrimination, and discordance between biological sex and gender identity (NEDA, 2018). Gay and bisexual men are also more likely to endure a spectrum of eating disorders for longer periods of time than heterosexual counterparts (NEDA, 2018). Individuals who have a strong sense of connectedness to the LGBT community are likely to have fewer eating disorders (NEDA, 2018).

Identifying and supporting the elimination of health disparities globally has been heavily criticized. In 2013, the WHO Secretariat developed a report acknowledging that, despite a lack of comprehensive global data, LGBT people face significant health challenges such as HIV, stress, shame, stigma, and violence (WHO, 2013). Furthermore, the report criticized medical school textbooks in Europe that identify homosexuality as a disease, the lack of trained health care professionals prepared to address unique health concerns for LGBT patients, the lack of comprehensive data on health disparities, and the lack of policies to support access to tailored care (WHO, 2013). However, the details of the report were met with protests by nations representing the African and the Eastern Mediterranean regions which resulted in the agenda item being removed from the meeting (Global Health Watch, 2018). Members cited numerous reasons why the topic should not be addressed in the meeting. Lee (2018) reports five main concerns that were raised by members, including: (1) LGBT individuals are choosing an "unhealthy lifestyle, which should not be encouraged," (2) focusing on LGBT health would result in "discrimination against others," (3) the topic of LGBT health is "too political," (4) "promoting LGBT issues is harmful to some countries' value systems," and (5) there is not enough proof, if any, that LGBT people face barriers in accessing health care (p. 18). Since that meeting, Lee (2018) reports that this topic has not been included in meetings.

In his own words

Steven M.
Coming out as a gay male can be challenging. I went to school in one of the most conservative states – North Carolina, and I recall one instance dating a guy who came from a conservative family. When they pulled him out of college for being gay, I could not fathom why anyone would do that. One night I went to meet him back in his hometown of Gastonia. I had to pick him up at work because his parents did not know. When I dropped him off, his parents and sister came barreling around the corner in their car and blocked my car with theirs. My heart was racing. I recall his father coming up to the driver's side window and saying that they don't want people of "my kind" around there.

Healthcare barriers

The biggest healthcare barrier that LGBTQ individuals face is discrimination (Mirza & Rooney, 2018). This discrimination can be intentional or unintentional, nevertheless it has the ability to cause physiological effects on the individual (Office of Disease Prevention and Health Promotion [ODPHP], 2019). In a survey conducted in 2017, 43.7 percent of LGBT persons reported that discrimination impacted their physical wellbeing (Singh & Durso, 2017).

A prominent example of healthcare discrimination for the LGBTQ community occurred when the United States experienced the AIDS epidemic in the 1980s. Much of this discrimination was due to society's disapproval of the associated sexual behaviors (Avert, 2019a). Nearly 40 years after the epidemic, LGBTQ individuals are still facing residual discrimination. Although there have been many achievements in treating and preventing HIV, the stigma that stemmed from the epidemic still affects LGBTQ persons today (Avert, 2019a). An example of current discriminatory policies/ practices can be seen in the U.S. Food and Drug Administration's (FDA) blood donor recommendations (2018). The FDA (2018) recommends that men who have sex with men must wait at least 12 months from their last sexual encounter to be eligible to donate blood. Human Rights Watch (2018) reports that transgender individuals have experienced providers suggesting simply praying that their lifestyle does not result in HIV and ultimately denying them access to PrEP (Pre-exposure Prophylaxis). LGBTQ individuals may not trust their healthcare providers with private details related to their health; this may discourage them from seeking out further necessary medical care. Winn (2012) recommends gay men discuss their health openly with their medical provider including topics on safe sex, hepatitis, fitness, substance use, mental health, STDs, cancer, tobacco, and HPV to learn about risks, diagnosis for health conditions, and recommended treatment plans, as needed.

Learn more

The National LGBT Cancer Network (2015) created an educational video called *Vanessa goes to the doctor* which demonstrates practices for creating medical offices that are LGBT inclusive. Watch the video online at www.youtube.com/watch?v=S3eDKf3PFRo.

Aside from both direct and indirect discrimination, there is also a lack of training of providers to meet the unique needs of the LGBT community. In a study conducted in 2012, 52% of medical students reported receiving no LGBT-competency training (Khalili, Leung, & Diamant, 2015). This statistic is particularly alarming since members of the LGBTQ community are disproportionately affected by mental illness, HIV, and the need to access hormonal therapy (Cohen, 2019).

Another barrier to healthcare services is the lack of financial stability. Specifically, members of the transgender community are disproportionately affected by homelessness and unemployment (Human Rights Watch, 2018). Due to this, it was reported that a quarter of transgender individuals were uninsured (Human Rights Watch, 2018).

> **Did you know?**
>
> OutCare Health (2018) compiles lists of LGBTQ competent healthcare providers. To learn more, visit www.outcarehealth.org/outlist/.

Best practices

Recognizing and educating on the topic of sexual orientation is important in eliminating stigma and discrimination. However, in Alabama, Louisiana, Mississippi, Oklahoma, South Carolina, and Texas there are specific laws in place, called "no promo homo," that prevent teaching on topics related to homosexuality (GLSEN, 2019). Laws vary and can range from not addressing homosexuality at all to only discussing the topic negatively (GLSEN, 2019). Sex education that is inclusive of LGBTQ explores the topic of sex and sexuality from a perspective that focuses on a wide range of behaviors across a spectrum and not solely on penile vaginal intercourse and pregnancy (Gowen & Winges-Yanez, 2014).

Key next steps to advance men's health

Healthy People 2020 is a set of recommendations for the United States to achieve positive health outcomes for all. Recommendations are based on the available research and data available at the time, across multiple topic areas. Specifically to improve the health of LGBT Americans, the guidelines acknowledge the lack of representative data (HealthyPeople. gov, 2019). Furthermore, the need for reducing violence targeting LGBT Americans and addressing health issues among older LGBT adults are also identified. Therefore, simply having access to data that accurately reflects the population is key to identifying prominent health issues and barriers to care. The Global Forum on MSM and HIV & OutRight Action International (2017) developed an inclusive global agenda for 2030 to improve the health of LGBT and intersex people (referred to as LGBTI) that includes nine distinct recommendations ranging from developing policies to protect LGBTI people from discrimination to collecting data that is representative of the population and preparing trained medical providers to address the health needs of LGBTI people. With targeted and sustained efforts, these recommendations address the challenges identified in this chapter and emphasize that better health outcomes are possible. Although there is no one answer as to how to move forward, it is evident that there is much work to be done to address the health needs of the LGBT population.

References

American Cancer Society. (2019). *Cancer facts for gay and bisexual men*. Retrieved from www. cancer.org/healthy/find-cancer-early/mens-health/cancer-facts-for-gay-and-bisexual-men. html#references

American Institute of Bisexuality. (2014a). *About Fritz Klein*. Retrieved from www. americaninstituteofbisexuality.org/fritz-klein

American Institute of Bisexuality. (2014b). *The Klein Sexual Orientation Grid*. Retrieved from www. americaninstituteofbisexuality.org/thekleingrid

Avert. (2019a). *HIV stigma and discrimination.* Retrieved from www.avert.org/professionals/hiv-social-issues/stigma-discrimination

Avert. (2019b). *Men who have sex with men (MSM), HIV and AIDS.* Retrieved from www.avert.org/professionals/hiv-social-issues/key-affected-populations/men-sex-men

Colapinto, J. (2000). *As Nature Made Him: The boy who was raised as a girl.* New York, NY: HarperCollins Publishers.

Centers for Disease Control and Prevention. (2017). *Syphilis and MSM [fact sheet].* Retrieved from www.cdc.gov/Std/syphilis/STDFact-MSM-Syphilis.htm

Centers for Disease Control and Prevention. (2019a). *HIV and African American gay and bisexual men.* Retrieved from www.cdc.gov/hiv/group/msm/bmsm.html

Centers for Disease Control and Prevention. (2019b). *HIV and gay and bisexual men.* Retrieved from www.cdc.gov/hiv/group/msm/index.html

Cohen, R. D. (2019). *Medical students push for more LGBT health training to address disparities.* Retrieved from www.npr.org/sections/health-shots/2019/01/20/68321 6767/medical-students-push-for-more-lgbt-health-training-to-address-disparities

Deveaux, F. (2016). *Counting the LGBT population: 6% of Europeans identify as LGBT.* Retrieved from https://daliaresearch.com/blog/counting-the-lgbt-population-6-of-europeans-identify-as-lgbt/

Erez, C., & Shenkman, G. (2016). Gay dads are happier: Subjective wellbeing among gay and heterosexual fathers. *Journal of GLBT Family Studies, 12*(5), 451–467. doi: 10.1080/1550428X.2015.1102668

Fenway Health. (2019). *About Fenway Health.* Retrieved from https://fenwayhealth.org/about/

Focus Features. (2019). *Milk.* Retrieved from www.focusfeatures.com/milk

Ganna, A., Verweij, K. J. H., Nivard, M. G., Maier, R., Wedow, R., Busch, A. S., … Zietsch, B. P. (2019). Large-scale GWAS reveals insights into the genetic architecture of same-sex sexual behavior. Science, *365*(6456). doi: 10.1126/science.aat7693

Gates, G. J. (2011). *How many people are lesbian, gay, bisexual, and transgender?* Retrieved from https://williamsinstitute.law.ucla.edu/wp-content/uploads/Gates-How-Many-People-LGBT-Apr-2011.pdf

Gender Spectrum. (2019). *The language of gender.* Retrieved from www.genderspectrum.org/the-language-of-gender/

GLAAD. (n.d.). *GLAAD media reference guide – Lesbian/Gay/Bisexual glossary of terms.* Retrieved from www.glaad.org/reference/lgbtq

GLSEN. (2019). *"No promo homo" laws & laws that prohibit enumeration by state.* Retrieved from www.glsen.org/policy-maps

Global, C. (2019). *Q&A: Director Hao Wu on coming out in a Chinese family.* Retrieved from http://chinafilminsider.com/qa-director-hao-wu-on-coming-out-in-a-chinese-family/

The Global Forum on MSM and HIV & OutRight Action International. (2017). *Agenda 2030 for LGBTI health and well-being.* Retrieved from https://msmgf.org/wp-content/uploads/2017/07/Agenda-2030-for-LGBTI-Health_July-2017.pdf

Global Health Watch. (2018). *EB133 May 2013.* Retrieved from www.ghwatch.org/who-watch/eb133

Gowen, L. K., & Winges-Yanez, N. (2014). Lesbian, gay, bisexual, transgender, queer, and questioning youths' perspectives of inclusive school-based sexuality education. *The Journal of Sex Research, 51*(7), 788–800. doi: 10.1080/00224499.2013.806648

Grinberg, E. (2019). *What the 'Q' in LGBTQ stands for, and other identity terms explained.* Retrieved from www.cnn.com/interactive/2019/06/health/lgbtq-explainer/

HealthyPeople.gov. (2019). *Lesbian, gay, bisexual, and transgender health.* Retrieved from www.healthypeople.gov/2020/topics-objectives/topic/lesbian-gay-bisexual-and-transgender-health#24

Human Rights Watch. (2018). *You don't want second best anti-LGBT discrimination in US health care.* Retrieved from www.hrw.org/report/2018/07/23/you-dont-want-second-best/anti-lgbt-discrimination-us-health-care

Human Rights Watch. (2019). *LGBT Rights.* Retrieved from www.hrw.org/topic/lgbt-rights

ILGA. (n.d.). *Maps: Sexual orientation laws.* Retrieved from https://ilga.org/maps-sexual-orientation-laws

interACT. (n.d.). *INTERSEX 101: Everything you want to know!* Retrieved from https://interactadvocates.org/wp-content/uploads/2017/03/INTERSEX101.pdf

Jones, J. M. (2017). *In U.S., 10.2% of LGBT adults now married to same-sex spouse.* Retrieved from https://news.gallup.com/poll/212702/lgbt-adults-married-sex-spouse.aspx

Khalili, J., Leung, L. B., & Diamant, A. L. (2015). Finding the perfect doctor: Identifying lesbian, gay, bisexual, and transgender-competent physicians. *American Journal of Public Health, 105*(6), 1114–1119. doi: 10.2105/ajph.2014.302448

Kinsey Institute. (2018). *The Kinsey Scale.* Retrieved from https://kinseyinstitute.org/research/publications/kinsey-scale.php

Lee, P. (2018). The demagogies of 'Lack': The WHO's ambivalence to the right to health of LGBT people. *Global Health Governance, 12*(1). Retrieved from http://blogs.shu.edu/ghg/files/2018/03/Spring-2018-Special-Issue.pdf#page=17

McCabe, S. E., West, B. T., Hughes, T. L., & Boyd, C. J. (2013). Sexual orientation and substance abuse treatment utilization in the United States: Results from a national survey. *Journal of Substance Abuse Treatment, 44*(1), 4–12. doi: 10.1016/j.jsat.2012.01.007.

Mirza, S. A., & Rooney, C. (2018). *Discrimination prevents LGBTQ people from accessing health care.* Retrieved from www.americanprogress.org/issues/lgbt/news/2018/01/18/445130/discrimination-prevents-lgbtq-people-accessing-health-care/

Movement Advancement Project. (2019). *Foster and adoption laws.* Retrieved from www.lgbtmap.org/equality-maps/foster_and_adoption_laws

Mustanski, B. S., Garofalo, R., & Emerson, E. M. (2010). Mental health disorders, psychological distress, and suicidality in a diverse sample of lesbian, gay, bisexual, and transgender youths. *American Journal of Public Health, 100*(12), 2426–2432. doi: 10.2105/AJPH.2009.178319

National Alliance on Mental Illness. (2019). *LGBTQ.* Retrieved from www.nami.org/find-support/lgbtq

National Eating Disorders Association. (2018). *Eating disorders in LGBTQ+ populations.* Retrieved from www.nationaleatingdisorders.org/learn/general-information/lgbtq

National Institute on Drug Abuse. (2017). *Substance use and SUDs in LGBTQ* populations.* Retrieved from www.drugabuse.gov/related-topics/substance-use-suds-in-lgbtq-populations

National LGBT Cancer Network. (2015). *Vanessa goes to the doctor.* Retrieved from www.youtube.com/watch?v=S3eDKf3PFRo

Newport, F. (2018). *In U.S., Estimate of LGBT population rises to 4.5%.* Retrieved from https://news.gallup.com/poll/234863/estimate-lgbt-population-rises.aspx

Obergefell v. Hodges, 135 S. Ct. 2584 (2015)

Office of Disease Prevention and Health Promotion. (2019). *Discrimination.* Retrieved from www.healthypeople.gov/2020/topics-objectives/topic/social-determinants-health/interventions-resources/discrimination

OutCare Health. (2018). *Find an LGBTQ competent healthcare provider.* Retrieved from www.outcarehealth.org/outlist/

Perrin, E., Hurley, S. M., Mattern, K., Flavin, L., & Pinderhughes, E. E. (2019). Barriers and stigma experienced by gay fathers and their children. *Pediatrics, 143*(2), e20180683. doi: https://doi.org/10.1542/peds.2018-0683

Perrin, E., Pinderhughes, E. E., Mattern, K., Hurley, S. M., & Newman, R. A. (2016). Experiences of children with gay fathers. *Clinical Pediatrics, 55*(14), 1305–1317. doi: 10.1177/0009922816632346

Pew Research. (2019). *Same-sex marriage around the world [Fact Sheet].* Retrieved from www.pewforum.org/fact-sheet/gay-marriage-around-the-world/

PFLAG. (2019). *About the Q.* Retrieved from https://pflag.org/blog/about-q

Sakas, M. E. (2018). *Colorado issues the state's first intersex birth certificate.* Retrieved from www.cpr.org/2018/09/22/colorado-issues-the-states-first-intersex-birth-certificate/

Singh, S., & Durso, L. E. (2017). *Widespread discrimination continues to shape LGBTQ people's lives in both subtle and significant ways.* Retrieved from www.americanprogres s.org/issues/lgbt/news/2017/05/02/429529/widespread-discrimination-continues-shape-lgbt-peoples-lives-subtle-significant-ways

UNAIDS (Joint United Nations Programme on HIV/AIDS). (2018). *UNAIDS Data 2018.* Retrieved from www.unaids.org/sites/default/files/media_asset/unaids-data-2018_en.pdf

United Nations. (n.d.). *Fact sheet: Intersex.* Retrieved from www.unfe.org/wp-content/uploads/2017/05/UNFE-Intersex.pdf

U.S. Food and Drug Administration. (2018). *Revised recommendations for reducing the risk of human immunodeficiency virus transmission by blood and blood products questions and answers.* Retrieved from www.fda.gov/vaccines-blood-biologics/blood-blood-products/revised-recommendations-reducing-risk-human-immunodeficiency-virus-transmission-blood-and-blood

visitreykjavik.is (2019). *LGBT Reykjavik.* Retrieved from https://visitreykjavik.is/city/lgbt-reykjavik

Ward, B. W., Dahlhamer, J. M., Galinsky, A. M., & Joestl, S. S. (2014). *Sexual orientation and health among U.S. adults: national health interview survey, 2013.* Retrieved from www.cdc.gov/nchs/data/nhsr/nhsr077.pdf.

Winn, R. J. (2012). *Ten things gay men should discuss with their healthcare provider.* GLMA (Gay & Lesbian Medical Association). Retrieved from https://falconhealth.org/wp-content/uploads/pdf/sexual-health-gay-men.pdf

Wolitski, R. J., Valdiserri, R., & Stall, R. (2007). *Overview of health disparities affecting gay and bisexual men* [PowerPoint slides]. Retrieved from https://apha.confex.com

World Health Organization. (2013). Executive Board Secretariat. *Improving the health and well-being of lesbian, gay, bisexual and transgender persons,* EB133/6. Retrieved from www.ghwatch.org/sites/www.ghwatch.org/files/B133-6_LGBT.pdf

World Health Organization. (2019). *Gender, equity and human rights.* Retrieved from www.who.int/gender-equity-rights/understanding/gender-definition/en/

7 Chronic diseases

Emil T. Chuck and Ledric D. Sherman

As the World Health Organization (WHO) acknowledges, non-communicable chronic illnesses are the leading category of illnesses responsible for mortality and morbidity worldwide (2019a). For the most part, modifying lifestyle behaviors and diet through cost-effective education and intervention coordinated with government leadership and support can reduce one's susceptibility. WHO (2019a) also estimates that 80% of premature heart disease, stroke, and diabetes could be prevented. Risk factors such as elevated blood glucose, elevated cholesterol, physical inactivity, obesity, high blood pressure, and an unhealthy diet impact individuals across the globe in staggering tolls as seen in Table 7.1 (WHO, 2019a). Furthermore, the Centers for Disease Control and Prevention (CDC) (2019) lists the top causes of death among adult men in the United States as heart disease, cancer, unintentional injuries, chronic lower respiratory disease, and stroke. In this chapter, we focus on the chronic illnesses of cardiovascular disease (CVD) and diabetes and emerging research that suggests associations of these diseases with other aspects of men's health.

Cardiovascular disease overview

CVD comprises an umbrella of pathologies that affect the heart and blood vessels in the brain. Peripheral vascular disease includes diseases of blood vessels outside of the heart and brain and is caused by the narrowing or blockage of blood vessels (The Johns Hopkins University, 2019a). Consisting of excessive fat, cholesterol, calcium, other proteins, and inflammation-responsive cells, plaque begins to line the smooth muscle of arteries, affecting the supply of oxygenated blood flow to target tissues. These blockages can result in damage to the heart, brain, or other organ tissues that can compromise their ability to function properly and can cause tissue damage or death. In addition, unstable plaques, including those caused by blood clots, can rupture and cause significant damage to tissues. CVD is the top cause of mortality and morbidity (WHO, 2019b), contributing to around 17 million deaths per year, 80% of which occur in low- to middle-income countries (Bovet & Paccaud, 2011). Experts report that by 2030, CVDs will account for almost 23.3 million deaths per year (WHO, 2019b). This burden is set to increase as a consequence of ageing populations and increasing levels of sedentary lifestyles, and obesity (Clar et al., 2017).

Cardiovascular disease preventative and early-stage treatment

In the early stages of CVD, lifestyle behavior modification remains the primary treatment. Healthy diet, routine exercise, and smoking cessation are fundamental to limiting, and possibly reversing, any damage. Nutritionists, dieticians, exercise physiologists, and

Table 7.1 Comparison of risk factors across the globe

Risk factor	Estimated world population affected
Elevated blood glucose	8.5% of adults aged 18 or older
High blood pressure	1.1 billion
Elevated cholesterol	39% of adults aged 25 or older
Physical inactivity	28% of adults aged 18 or older, 2016; 80% of adolescents aged 11–17
Overweight/obesity	39% of men and 39% of women aged 18 or older
Unhealthy diet	1.7 million deaths attributed to low fruit and vegetable consumption

kinesiologists may be consulted to address questions and develop individualized meal plans where appropriate. Understanding and addressing psychological, cultural, and societal factors can affect someone's success in maintaining those lifestyle changes.

Cardiovascular disease treatment and diagnosis

Undiagnosed and/or untreated patients will likely experience symptoms such as chest pain, shortness of breath, peripheral neuropathy, blurred vision, loss of energy, and increased urination. However, patients often discover their illness with a sudden incident such as a myocardial infarction (also referred to as a heart attack) or stroke. Surgical interventions include delivery of drug-eluting stents in blocked arteries to maintain blood flow to critical tissues (including the heart and brain) while reducing any subsequent blockages due to plaque formation and calcification or blood clots. In situations where cardiac function is severely compromised, ventricular assist devices are surgically implanted.

Prescription interventions

In more severe cases, medications may be prescribed to lower cholesterol, reduce blood pressure, and prevent blood clots. Statins are most commonly prescribed and clinically studied. Statins have clinically demonstrated their efficacy in reducing outcomes for people with CVD and those who have had a stroke or heart attack (Fogoros, 2019a). While lifestyle management remains the most cost-effective treatment for high blood pressure, prescription medication assistance is often needed for addressing more inherent risk factors (such as male sex and family history). In general, five major drug families have been clinically effective. These include diuretics (also called water pills) to increase the amount of sodium and water excreted from the body, thus reducing blood pressure by reducing fluid volume in the circulation; beta-blockers which reduce the effects of adrenaline in the body, resulting in a slower heart rate and lower stress in the heart and arteries; calcium-channel blockers which dilate the arteries and sometimes slow heart rate to reduce blood pressure; angiotension-converting enzyme (ACE) inhibitors which dilate the arteries to lower blood pressure; and, angiotension-II-receptor blockers (ARBs) which also dilate the arteries to lower blood pressure (Fogoros, 2019b). Depending on the severity of hypertension (also referred to as high blood pressure), a combination therapy of drugs involving two or more families may also be considered and prescribed (American Heart Association, 2017). Anti-thrombotics may be prescribed to prevent blood clots. They are generally classified as either anti-coagulant or anti-platelet drugs. Anticoagulants, such as heparin and warfarin, act on reducing the formation of fibrin during the clotting process. In contrast, anti-platelet drugs such as aspirin prevent platelets from clumping to form clots (American Society of Hematology, 2019). Additional research in diagnostics focuses on identification of more biomarkers that more clearly informs clinicians and patients on identifying early-stage disease to implement preventative strategies and care (Srikanthan, Feyh, Visweshwar, Shapiro, & Sodhi, 2016).

CVD and diabetes share similar risk factors of physical inactivity, obesity, and high blood pressure (American Heart Association, 2015). In addition, a risk factor for CVD (The Johns Hopkins University, 2019b; Katsiki, Wierzbicki, & Mikhailidis, 2015) and a possible complication of diabetes is erectile dysfunction, commonly referred to as ED.

Diabetes overview

More than 100 million adults in the United States are living with diabetes or prediabetes, which is a condition that, if not treated, often leads to type 2 diabetes within five years (CDC, 2017). In the United States, 30.3 million people (or 9.4% of the population) have diabetes, approximately 23.1 million of whom are diagnosed and 7.2 million are undiagnosed (CDC, 2017). Slightly more men (15.3 million) have diabetes than women (14.9 million) in the United States (CDC, 2017). According to the International Diabetes Federation (IDF) (2017), globally, there are more deaths attributable to diabetes in women (2.1 million) than in men (1.8 million). However, North America and the Caribbean are the only regions where there are more deaths attributable to diabetes in men than women (IDF, 2017). In sub-Saharan Africa, it is estimated that 15.5 million adults aged 20–79 years of age have diabetes, with the highest prevalence between the ages of 55 and 64 (IDF, 2017). Furthermore, some of Africa's most populous countries have the highest numbers of people with diabetes, including Ethiopia (2.6 million), South Africa (1.8 million), Democratic Republic of Congo (1.7 million), and Nigeria (1.7 million) (IDF, 2017). Diabetes-attributable mortality is 1.6 times higher in women (185,049) compared to men (113,110) (IDF, 2017). This may be because men are more likely to succumb to death from other causes, such as armed conflict.

On the continent of Europe, it is estimated that the number of people with diabetes is 58 million, including 22 million undiagnosed cases (IDF, 2017). Turkey has the highest age-adjusted comparative prevalence and the third highest number of people with diabetes in Europe (6.7 million), after Germany (7.5 million) and the Russian Federation (8.5 million) (IDF, 2017). In Europe, there are more deaths due to diabetes in women compared to men (413,807 and 279,543, respectively) (IDF, 2017). This is due to the higher number of diabetes cases in women (30.8 million) than men (28.8 million) and the higher number of women in the population (350.1 million) than men (321.4 million) (IDF, 2017).

In the Middle East and North African region, it is estimated that approximately 38.7 million people are living with diabetes (IDF, 2017). Countries with the highest age-adjusted comparative diabetes prevalence in the Middle East are Saudi Arabia (17.7%), Egypt (17.3%), and the United Arab Emirates (17.3%), and the countries with the largest number of adults aged 20–79 years with diabetes are Egypt (8.2 million), Pakistan (7.5 million), and Iran (5.0 million) (IDF, 2017). There is more mortality due to diabetes among women at 190,887 than among men at 127,148 (IDF, 2017). The reason is probably due to the higher number of women with diabetes (women: 1.95 million; men: 1.91 million) and, conceivably, men are more likely to succumb to death from other causes (IDF, 2017).

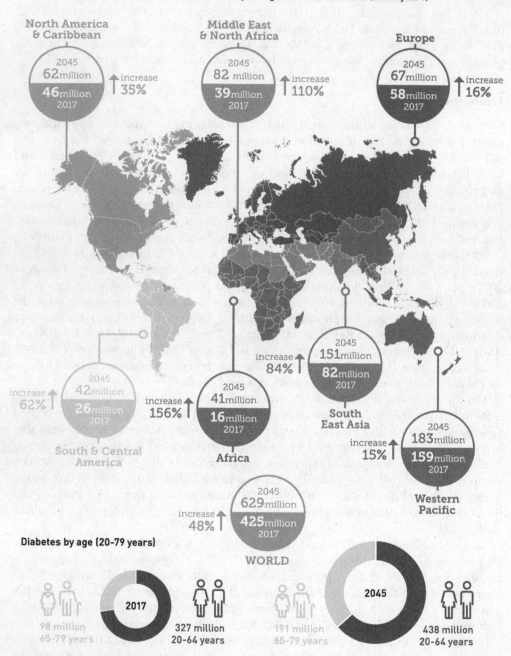

Figure 7.1 Number of people with diabetes worldwide and per regions in 2017 and 2045 (20–79 years).

Source: International Diabetes Federation (2017).

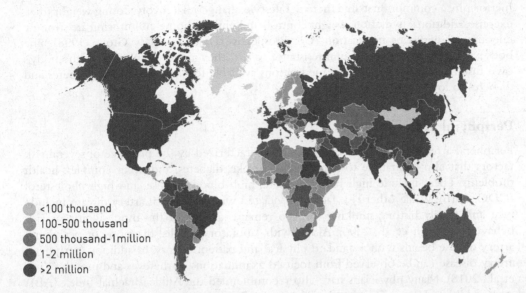

Figure 7.2 Estimated total numbers of adults (20–79 years) living with diabetes in 2017.
Source: International Diabetes Federation (2017).

After investigating the diabetes numbers across the globe, one item to note is that the number of deaths from diabetes among U.S. men is higher than for men who reside in other countries around the world.

Types of diabetes

Typically, the body breaks down the carbohydrates you eat into sugar, or glucose, that it uses for energy. Insulin is a hormone that the body needs to get glucose from the bloodstream into the cells of the body. Although there are many similarities between type 1 and type 2 diabetes, the cause of each is very different. In type 1 diabetes, the body does not produce insulin. Type 2 diabetes is the more common form of diabetes where the body does not use insulin properly. While some people can control their blood glucose levels with healthy eating and exercise, others may need medication or insulin to help manage it. With the help of insulin therapy and other treatments, everyone can learn to manage their condition and live long healthy lives. According to the American Diabetes Association (ADA 2019a), the symptoms for type 1 and type 2 diabetes include frequent urination, feeling thirsty often, feeling hungry even when you are eating, extreme fatigue, blurry vision, cuts or bruises that are slow to heal, and tingling, pain or numbness in your hands and feet. A diagnosis for type 2 diabetes is confirmed with a simple blood test called an A1C, with a result higher than 6.5% (ADA, 2019b)

Adults who are newly diagnosed with type 1 diabetes may have symptoms similar to type 2 diabetes, and this overlap between types can be confusing. Some people with type 2 diabetes have symptoms that are so mild that they often go unnoticed. Early detection and treatment of diabetes can decrease the risk of developing the complications of diabetes, such as blindness, kidney disease, ED, and amputations. Patients who have elevated high blood glucose who may be at risk of developing type 2 diabetes are typically given metformin, a common first-line therapy. Lifestyle changes that involve losing weight (diet, exercise, additional hydration, weight control) and glucose home-monitoring are strongly encouraged with this medication (UK Prospective Diabetes Study Group, 1998). The body's tissues may develop insulin resistance so that they are less responsive to the body's own insulin. There are additional medications available for patients with prediabetes and diabetes to lower blood glucose levels.

Peripheral artery disease

Peripheral artery disease is a serious disease characterized by the presence of several risk factors that also contribute to heart disease, stroke, diabetes, and other complex health problems. These include high blood pressure, high blood glucose, and high cholesterol (CDC, 2016). While other risk factors associated with peripheral artery disease include race and family history, smoking tobacco remains as one of the most significant risk behaviors (Hirsch et al., 2006). Along with laboratory results, diagnosis of peripheral artery disease begins with a standard physical and patient history. In addition, peripheral artery disease can be observed from focused examinations of the eyes and mouth (Yang et al., 2018). Many physicians have also recommended the Ankle-Brachial Index (ABI) as an additional screening test, though systematic reviews come to mixed conclusions (Alahdab et al., 2015; Hennion & Siano, 2013). The ABI screening is a comparison of the blood pressures of the arms and legs (Stanford Medicine, 2019). Finally, swelling of the feet, ankles, and legs, along with ED, are also associated with peripheral artery disease. Progression of the disease is often associated with decreased walking distance without pain or difficulty (Abdulhannan, Russell, & Homer-Vanniasinkam, 2012).

Development of the disease is generally invisible since symptoms may not be apparent. For some, the initial symptoms may include pain or cramping in the legs or thighs during or after exercise (Cleveland Clinic, n.d.). Numbness and weakness may also be observed. However, many with peripheral artery disease may present no symptoms even with severely blocked peripheral vessels (Cleveland Clinic, n.d.).

Did you know?

The National Diabetes and Education Program (NDEP) works collaboratively with its partners at the federal, state, and local levels to improve the treatment and outcomes for people with diabetes, promote early diagnosis, and prevent or delay the onset of type 2 diabetes (National Institutes of Health, n.d.). Learn more at www.niddk.nih.gov/health-information/communication-programs/ndep.

Learn more

The ADA, AHA, and AARP have teamed up to create resources available for home delivery (referred to as boxes) that contain useful health tools and resources for those with diabetes or CVD (AARP, 2019). To learn more, visit https://letsbewell.com/pages/about-us.

Personal assessment

Do you think you're at risk for diabetes? The ADA (2019c) offers an online risk test for type 2 diabetes at https://diabetes.org/risk-test.

In his own words

Stephen D, 40. Diagnosed with diabetes, high triglycerides, and high cholesterol at age 39

The only reason that I even bothered to get it checked out was because my wife was feeling sick and wanted to go to the doctor and I figured since I was already at the doctor … .

Looking back I had a lot of the telltale symptoms [of diabetes]. I was drinking excessive amounts of water, and then excessively urinating, and I had rapid weight loss. But none of those bothered me. I figured I'd just rub some dirt on it and I'd be fine. Even when I went to donate platelets and they told me that my donation was garbage and unusable [because of the high fat content] I didn't feel the need to get checked. I went with my wife to the initial doctor's appointments, and information about diet was directed to her.

Masculinity and chronic health issues in men

In the United States and most countries in the world, males are more likely than females to die in their first year of life and at every age across the remainder of the life course (Williams, 2003). Distinct and persistent evidence suggests that health practices have a vital role in the etiology of most of the preeminent causes of death among men (Courtenay, 2000, 2003; Creighton & Oliffe, 2010; Robertson, 2008; Thorpe et al., 2013). An aspect that can contribute to the numbers of men worldwide in relation to help-seeking, as well as disease management, is male masculinity. Masculinity is defined in various ways that range by race, ethnicity, class, sexual identity, disability status, and other factors, but are centered on a common association in the category of *a man* (Hurtado & Sinha, 2008). Preceding research examining the relationship between masculinity and health was overshadowed by the premise that biological sex played an essential role in determining health behaviors, however, scholars have paid expanding attention to the health ramifications of gendered expectations and normative gender roles in men's health (Broom & Tovey, 2009; Robertson, 2007). Men will often prefer to jeopardize their physical health and well-being rather than be linked with traits they or others may perceive as feminine (Bruce, Roscigno, & McCall, 1998; Evans, Frank, Oliffe, & Gregory, 2011; Messerschmidt, 2013).

Masculinity has chiefly been operationalized and considered as a static factor that resides entirely in each man's respective psychology (Courtenay, 2002), but masculinity is often signified by beliefs and behaviors that transition over time and that are applied in everyday social and cultural patterns, practices, and relations (Courtenay, 2002;

Moynihan, 1998; Smiler, 2006). Throughout life, the stressors correlated with feelings and notions about men's behavior, economic opportunities, and social marginalization can precisely and incidentally contribute to men having poor health behaviors and high rates of morbidity from preventable ailments (Williams, 2003). Progressively, masculinity is being conceptualized and framed to be best inferred to or known in the context of social and cultural factors (Creighton & Oliffe, 2010; Robertson, 2006). Masculinity is not something that commonly exists in the minds of individual men; masculinity is learned, shaped, and reproduced through interpersonal associations with other men and women and within numerous settings such as neighborhoods, schools, and faith-based organizations (Creighton & Oliffe, 2010). While masculinity is considered to be a meaningful consideration of men's health, the study of men's health and well-being has not always hypothesized men as gendered beings (Evans et al., 2011; Kimmel, 2000; Kimmel, Hearn, & Connell, 2005).

Emerging issues

Tailored education for men on a variety of chronic health issues is important. However, there are insufficient reports on health information being provided to, for example, Australian men in male-specific settings that offer health promotion opportunities (such as Men's Sheds, Men's Health Nights) (Golding, Brown, Foley, Harvey, & Gleeson, 2007; Morgan, Hayes, Williamson, & Ford, 2007; Verrinder & Denner, 2000). Men's inadequate health knowledge (Courtenay 1998, 2000; Evans et al., 2007) is also "associated with … unhealthy behaviors" (Courtenay, 2003, p. 14). One example of how to overcome these gaps is through the MensLine Australia (n.d.), which is a national hotline for men to contact for questions and support in their relationships, with substance use, violence, and overall health. In the United States, discussions of men's health have focused on their underutilization of preventative care and possible causes, influenced by health-related beliefs and behaviors, but not the role of health literacy (Courtenay, 2003; Holland, 2005).

An aspect of disease management that should be considered for continued improvement among male patients is health literacy, particularly among those with diabetes. Patients' health literacy may be significantly worse than their general literacy skills because of unfamiliar medical vocabulary and concepts (Powell, Hill, & Clancy, 2007). The Institute of Medicine (2004) has previously defined low health literacy as a lack of the capacity to obtain, process, and understand basic health information and services needed to make appropriate health decisions, and has been considered as a potential barrier to improving health outcomes.

Patients with inadequate health literacy may also have difficulty performing relatively simple yet crucial tasks, such as comprehending medication labels and appointment slips (American Medical Association, 2009). Low health literacy is associated with poor disease-related knowledge and self-management strategies, worse self-reported health status, poor adherence with treatment, a 30% to 50% increased risk of hospitalization, and higher annual health care costs (Powell et al., 2007). In particular, patients with diabetes, who must engage in constant self-management, must have adequate health literacy to apply the requisite knowledge, decision-making skills, and problem-solving skills for effective diabetes management (Fransen, von Wagner, & Essink-Bot, 2012).

While there is a developing literature on gender and health, insufficient consideration has been given to the function of gender in health literacy. This is notwithstanding the inflation of public health crusades and programs advocating for extensive community awareness and behavior modification about risk factors, particularly those pertaining to chronic disease (Health Council of Canada, 2007; WHO, 2017; WHO Commission on Social Determinants of Health, 2008). Gender has previously been defined as "a dynamic set of socially constructed relationships embedded in everyday interaction, rather than a simple attribute of individuals" (Emslie & Hunt, 2008, p. 808). Health outcomes throughout countries mirror gender-based patterns as well as occupational and socio-economic groups, relevant to men's attitudes and practices to health concerns (such as seeking medical attention), and susceptibility for chronic ailments (such as nutrition and obesity) (Courtenay, 2000; DeSouza & Ciclitira, 2005; Mahalik, Burns, & Syzdek, 2007; Muenning, Lubetkin, Jia, & Franks, 2006; Murray, Lopez, World Health Organization, World Bank, & Harvard School of Public Health, 1996; Roos, Prättäläb, & Koski, 2001; Smith, 2008; Smith, Braunack-Mayer, & Wittert, 2006).

The threat of complications from diabetes, for example, is higher among patients with low health literacy, as they are less likely to have suitable knowledge of diabetes and related self-care activities than are those with appropriate health literacy (Al Sayah, Majumdar, Williams, Robertson, & Johnson, 2013). Previous research efforts have proposed a variety of interventions to enhance health outcomes and diminish the health disparity associated with low health literacy. The strategies recurrently recommended to healthcare providers include, but are not limited to, implementing health literacy policy changes, advancing the usability of health information by using plain language, improving the listening and speaking among patients, focusing on actions, limiting the number of messages, acknowledging cultural differences, supplementing instructions with pictures, and checking that patients understand (Kim & Lee, 2016; The Office of Disease Prevention and Health Promotion, 2015).

Future research

Men often use health patterns and practices in daily interactions to assist them in negotiating social power and social status, and these health practices can either impair or enhance their health (Courtenay & Keeling, 2000). How men conceptualize about and exhibit an image of themselves as men and respond to gendered social norms and pressures is often implied in explanations of men's premature death due to stress and unhealthy behaviors (such as reckless driving, alcohol and drug abuse, risky sexual behavior, high-risk sports, and leisure activities) (Griffith, Gunter, & Allen, 2011; Peterson, 2009). Therefore, there is an enduring need for health research and practice that is gender conscious in regard to men's lives and to discern masculinities with regard to health and illness (Evans et al., 2011), which may come through comprehending the relationship between masculinity and differing aspects of men's health.

Investigating prior characterized attributes of masculinity among men diagnosed with diabetes will also permit health professionals and researchers to comprehend how racial identity and cultural tradition can affect the development of social norms regarding the acceptance and continual practice of healthy diabetes management behaviors among family members, friends of the same gender, and friends of the opposite gender (Jack, Tyson, Jack, & Sims, 2010).

Future gender-based diabetes research efforts among men across the globe should consider examining gender role conflict. Investigating the benefits and costs for men and others in their immediate social support network (such as a spouse, partner, family) for both conforming and not conforming to conventional gender role norms would be advantageous to men across the globe and their families (Mahalik et al., 2003; Porche, 2007). Ultimately, examining aspects of gender from a male worldview would help multiple fields of interest to identify the role of masculinity in shaping how international men, their families, and significant others cooperatively are able to effectively manage chronic health issues.

References

AARP. (2019). *The Let's Be Well story.* Retrieved from https://letsbewell.com/pages/about-us

Abdulhannan, P., Russell, D. A., & Homer-Vanniasinkam, S. (2012). Peripheral arterial disease: A literature review. *British Medical Bulletin, 104*(1), 21–39. https://doi.org/10.1093/bmb/lds027

Alahdab, F., Wang, A. T., Elraiyah, T. A., Malgor, R. D., Rizvi, A. Z., Lane, M. A., … Murad, M. H. (2015). A systematic review for the screening for peripheral arterial disease in asymptomatic patients. *Journal of Vascular Surgery, 61*(3, Supplement), 42S–53S. https://doi.org/10.1016/j.jvs.2014.12.008

Al Sayah, F., Majumdar, S. R., Williams, B., Robertson, S., & Johnson, J. A. (2013). Health literacy and health outcomes in diabetes: A systematic review. *Journal of General Internal Medicine, 28*(3), 444–452.

American Diabetes Association. (2019a). *Diabetes symptoms.* Retrieved from www.diabetes.org/diabetes/type-2/symptoms

American Diabetes Association. (2019b). *Understanding A1C.* Retrieved from www.diabetes.org/a1c

American Diabetes Association. (2019c). *Our 60-second type 2 diabetes risk test.* Retrieved from www.diabetes.org/risk-test

American Heart Association. (2015). *Top 10 myths about cardiovascular disease.* Retrieved from www.heart.org/en/health-topics/consumer-healthcare/what-is-cardiovascular-disease/top-10-myths-about-cardiovascular-disease

American Heart Association. (2017). *Highlights from the 2017 Guideline for the prevention, detection, evaluation and management of high blood pressure in adults.* Retrieved from https://healthmetrics.heart.org/wp-content/uploads/2017/11/Highlights-from-the-2017-Guideline.pdf

American Medical Association. (2009) Health literacy: report of the Council on Scientific Affairs. *Journal of the American Medical Association, 28*, 552–557.

American Society of Hematology. (2019). *Antithrombotic therapy.* Retrieved from www.hematology.org/About/History/50-Years/1523.aspx

Bovet, P., & Paccaud, F. (2011). Cardiovascular disease and the changing face of global public health: A focus on low and middle income countries. *Public Health Reviews, 33*(2), 397–415. https://doi.org/10.1007/BF03391643

Broom, A., & Tovey, P. (Eds.). (2009). *Men's Health: Body, identity and social context.* Chichester: Wiley-Blackwell.

Bruce, M. A., Roscigno, V. J., & McCall, P. L. (1998). Structure, context, and agency in the reproduction of black-on-black violence. *Theoretical Criminology, 2*(1), 29–55.

Centers for Disease Control and Prevention. (2016). *Peripheral Arterial Disease (PAD) [Fact Sheet].* Retrieved from www.cdc.gov/dhdsp/data_statistics/fact_sheets/fs_pad.htm

Centers for Disease Control and Prevention. (2017). *National Diabetes Statistics Report, 2017.* Retrieved from www.cdc.gov/diabetes/pdfs/data/statistics/national-diabetes-statistics-report.pdf

Centers for Disease Control and Prevention. (2019). *FastStats.* Retrieved from www.cdc.gov/nchs/fastats/mens-health.htm

Clar, C., Al-Khudairy, L., Loveman, E., Kelly, S. A., Hartley, L., Flowers, N., … Rees, K. (2017). Low glycaemic index diets for the prevention of cardiovascular disease. *Cochrane Database of Systematic Reviews,* (7). https://doi.org/10.1002/14651858.CD004467.pub3

Cleveland Clinic. (n.d.). *Peripheral Arterial Disease (PAD)*. Retrieved from https://my.clevelandclinic.org/health/diseases/17357-peripheral-artery-disease-pad

Courtenay, W. (1998). College men's health: An overview and a call to action. *Journal of American College Health, 46*(6), 279–290.

Courtenay, W. (2000). Constructions of masculinity and their influence on men's well-being: A theory of gender and health. *Social Science and Medicine, 50*, 1385–1401.

Courtenay, W. (2002). A global perspective on the field of men's health: An editorial. *International Journal of Men's Health, 1*, 1–13.

Courtenay, W. H. (2003). Key determinants of the health and well-being of men and boys. *International Journal of Men's Health, 2*, 1–30.

Courtenay, W. H., & Keeling, R. P. (2000). Men, gender, and health: Toward an interdisciplinary approach. *Journal of American College Health, 48*(6), 1–4.

Creighton, G., & Oliffe, J. L. (2010). Theorising masculinities and men's health: A brief history with a view to practice. *Health Sociology Review, 19*(4), 409–418.

DeSouza, P., & Ciclitira, K. E. (2005). Men and dieting: A qualitative analysis. *Journal of Health Psychology, 10*(6), 793–804.

Emslie, C., & Hunt, K. (2008). The weaker sex? Exploring lay understandings of gender and differences in life expectancy: a qualitative study. *Social Science and Medicine, 67*, 808–816.

Evans, J., Frank, B., Oliffe, J. L., & Gregory, D. J. (2011). Health, Illness, Men and Masculinities (HIMM): A theoretical framework for understanding men and their health. *Journal of Men's Health, 8*(1), 7–15.

Evans, R., Edwards, A. G. K., Elwyn, G., Watson, E., Grol, R., Brett, J., & Austoker, J. (2007). 'It's a Maybe Test': Men's experiences of prostate specific antigen testing in primary care. *British Journal of General Practice, 57*, 303–310.

Fogoros, R. (2019a). *How different drugs can help lower your cholesterol*. Retrieved from www.verywellhealth.com/drugs-for-cholesterol-and-triglycerides-1745831

Fogoros, R. (2019b). *Your complete guide to hypertension drugs*. Retrieved from www.verywellhealth.com/hypertension-drugs-1745989

Fransen, M. P., von Wagner, C., & Essink-Bot, M. L. (2012). Diabetes self-management in patients with low health literacy: Ordering findings from literature in a health literacy framework. *Patient Education and Counseling, 88*(1), 44–53.

Golding, B., Brown, M., Foley, A., Harvey, J. & Gleeson, L. (2007). *Men's sheds in Australia: Learning through community contexts*. Retrieved from www.ncver.edu.au/research-and-statistics/publications/all-publications/mens-sheds-in-australia-learning-through-community-contexts

Griffith, D. M., Gunter, K., & Allen, J. O. (2011). Male gender role strain as a barrier to African American men's physical activity. *Health Education Behavior, 38*, 482–491.

Health Council of Canada. (2007). *Why health care renewal matters: Learning from Canadians with chronic health conditions*. Retrieved from https://healthcouncilcanada.ca files/2.20-Outcomes2FINAL.pdf

Hennion, D. R., & Siano, K. A. (2013). Diagnosis and treatment of Peripheral Arterial Disease. *American Family Physician, 88*(5), 306–310.

Hirsch, A. T., Haskal, Z. J., Hertzer, N. R., Bakal, C. W., Creager, M. A., Halperin, J. L., … Vascular Disease Foundation. (2006). ACC/AHA 2005 Practice guidelines for the management of patients with peripheral arterial disease (lower extremity, renal, mesenteric, and abdominal aortic). *Circulation, 113*(11), e463–654. doi: 0.1161/CIRCULATIONAHA.106.174526

Holland, D. J. (2005). Sending men the message about preventive care: an evaluation of communication strategies. *International Journal of Men's Health, 4*(2), 97–114.

Hurtado, A., & Sinha, M. (2008). More than men: Latino feminist masculinities and intersectionality. *Sex Roles, 59*(5–6), 337–349. doi: 10.1007/s11199-008-9405-7

Institute of Medicine. (2004). *Health Literacy: A prescription to end confusion*. Washington, DC: The National Academies Press. https://doi.org/10.17226/10883.

International Diabetes Federation. (2017). *IDF Diabetes Atlas 8th edition*. Retrieved from www.idf.org/e-library/epidemiology-research/diabetes-atlas/134-idf-diabetes-atlas-8th-edition.html

Jack, L., Jr., Tyson, T., Jack, N., & Sims, M. (2010). A gender-centered ecological framework targeting Black men living with diabetes: Integrating a "masculinity" perspective in diabetes management and education research. *American Journal of Men's Health, 4,* 7–15.

The Johns Hopkins University. (2019a). *Peripheral Vascular Disease.* Retrieved from www.hopkinsmedicine.org/health/conditions-and-diseases/peripheral-vascular-disease

The Johns Hopkins University. (2019b). *Special heart risks for men.* Retrieved from www.hopkinsmedicine.org/health/wellness-and-prevention/special-heart-risks-for-men

Katsiki, N., Wierzbicki, A. S., & Mikhailidis, D. P. (2015). Erectile dysfunction and coronary heart disease. *Current Opinion in Cardiology, 30*(4), 416–421. doi: 10.1097/HCO.0000000000000174

Kim, S. H., & Lee, A. (2016). Health-literacy-sensitive diabetes self-management interventions: A systematic review and meta-analysis. *Worldviews on Evidence-Based Nursing, 13*(4), 324–333.

Kimmel, M. (2000). *The Gendered Society.* New York: Oxford University Press.

Kimmel, M., Hearn J., & Connell, R. W. (2005). *Handbook on Studies on Men & Masculinities.* Thousand Oaks, CA: Sage.

Mahalik, J. R., Burns, S. M., & Syzdek, M. (2007). Masculinity and perceived normative health behaviors as predictors of men's health behaviors. *Social Science and Medicine, 64,* 2201–2209.

Mahalik, J. R., Locke, B., Ludlow, L., Diemer, M., Scott, R. P. J., Gottfried, M., & Freitas, G. (2003). Development of the conformity to masculine norms inventory. *Psychology of Men & Masculinity, 4,* 3–25.

MensLine Australia. (n.d.). *About MensLine Australia.* Retrieved from https://mensline.org.au/about-us/

Messerschmidt, J. (2013). *Crime as Structured Action: Doing masculinities, race, class, sexuality and crime.* 2nd ed. Plymouth, UK: Rowman & Littlefield.

Morgan, M., Hayes, R., Williamson, M., & Ford, C. (2007). Men's sheds: A community approach to promoting mental health and well-being. *International Journal of Mental Health Promotion, 9*(3), 50–54.

Moynihan, C. (1998). Theories in health care and research. *British Medical Journal, 317,* 1072–1075.

Muenning, P., Lubetkin, E., Jia, H., & Franks, P. (2006). Gender and the burden of disease attributable to obesity. *American Journal of Public Health, 96*(9), 1662–1668.

Murray, C. J. L., Lopez, A. D., World Health Organization, World Bank, & Harvard School of Public Health. (1996). *The Global Burden of Disease: A comprehensive assessment of mortality and disability from diseases, injuries, and risk factors in 1990 and projected to 2020.* Cambridge, MA: Harvard University Press. Retrieved from https://apps.who.int/iris/bitstream/handle/10665/41864/0965546608_eng.pdf?sequence=1&isAllowed=y

National Institutes of Health. (n.d.). *National Diabetes Education Program.* Retrieved from www.niddk.nih.gov/health-information/communication-programs/ndep

The Office of Disease Prevention and Health Promotion. (2015). *Quick guide to health literacy.* Retrieved from https://health.gov/communication/literacy/quickguide/

Peterson, A. (2009). Future research agenda in men's health. In A. Tovey & P. Bloom (Eds.), *Men's Health: Body, identity and social context* (pp. 202–213). Chichester, UK: Wiley-Blackwell.

Porche, D. (2007). A call for American Journal of Men's Health. *American Journal of Men's Health, 1,* 5–7.

Powell, C. K., Hill, E. G., & Clancy, D. E. (2007). The relationship between health literacy and diabetes knowledge and readiness to take health actions. *The Diabetes Educator, 33*(1), 144–151.

Robertson, S. (2006). 'I've been like a coiled spring this last week': Embodied masculinity and health. *Sociology of Health & Illness, 28*(4), 433–456.

Robertson, S. (2007). *Understanding Men and Health: Masculinities, identities and well-being.* McGraw Hill Open University Press: UK.

Robertson, S. (2008). *Theories of masculinities and health seeking practices.* Paper presented at the "Nowhere Man" Men's Health Seminar, Stormont, Ireland. Retrieved from www.mensproject.org/issues/stevespeech.pdf

Roos, G., Prättäläb, R., & Koski, K. (2001). Men, masculinity and food: Interviews with Finnish carpenters and engineers. *Appetite, 37,* 47–56. doi: 10.1006/appe.2001.0409

Smiler, A. P. (2006). Introduction to manifestations of masculinity. *Sex Roles, 55,* 585–587. doi: 10.1007/s11199-006-9114-z

Smith, J. A. (2008). The men's health policy contexts in Australia, the UK and Ireland: Advancement or abandonment? *Journal of Critical Public Health, 19*(3–4), 427–440.

Smith, J. A., Braunack-Mayer, A., & Wittert, G. (2006). What do we know about men's help seeking and health service use? *Medical Journal of Australia, 184*(2), 81–83.

Srikanthan, K., Feyh, A., Visweshwar, H., Shapiro, J. I., & Sodhi, K. (2016). Systematic review of metabolic syndrome biomarkers: A panel for early detection, management, and risk stratification in the West Virginian population. *International Journal of Medical Sciences, 13*(1), 25–38. https://doi.org/10.7150/ijms.13800

Stanford Medicine. (2019). *Introduction to measuring the ankle brachial index.* Retrieved from https://stanfordmedicine25.stanford.edu/the25/ankle.html

Thorpe, R. J., Wilson-Frederick, S. M., Bowie, J. V., Coa, K., Clay, O. J., LaVeist, T. A., & Whitfield, K. E. (2013). Health behaviors and all-cause mortality in African American men. *American Journal of Men's Health, 7*(suppl.4), 8S–18S.

UK Prospective Diabetes Study Group. (1998). Effect of intensive blood-glucose control with metformin on complications in overweight patients with type 2 diabetes (UKPDS 34). *Lancet, 352*(9131), 854–865.

Verrinder, A., & Denner, B. (2000). The success of men's health nights and health sessions. *Australian Journal of Rural Health, 8,* 81–86.

Williams, D. R. (2003). The health of men: Structured inequalities and opportunities. *American Journal of Public Health, 92,* 588–597.

World Health Organization Commission on Social Determinants of Health. (2008). *Closing the Gap in a Generation: Health equity through action on social determinants of health.* Geneva: WHO.

World Health Organization. (2017). *Global Strategy on Diet, Physical Activity and Health.* Geneva: WHO.

World Health Organization. (2019a). *Noncommunicable diseases (NCD).* Retrieved from www.who.int/gho/ncd/en/

World Health Organization. (2019b). *NCD mortality and morbidity.* Retrieved from www.who.int/gho/ncd/mortality_morbidity/en/

Yang, S., Zhao, L. S., Cai, C., Shi, Q., Wen, N., & Xu, J. (2018). Association between periodontitis and peripheral artery disease: A systematic review and meta-analysis. *BMC Cardiovascular Disorders, 18*(1), 141. https://doi.org/10.1186/s12872-018-0879-0

Part III

Relationships

8 Mental health

*Salvatore J. Giorgianni, Jr., Armin Brott, Susan A. Milstein,
and Diana Karczmarczyk*

Mental health issues can be especially problematic for society. Defining exactly what constitutes deliberate unlawful behavior, immorality, or conduct resulting from involuntary brain dysfunction is often challenging. Unlike most medical illnesses, there are usually few specific objective and measurable factors by which to establish a diagnosis. Unlike most physical health disorders, mental health disorders are frequently stigmatized. People may be labeled crazy, leading to a person being ostracized, ashamed and reluctant to seek help.

For men and boys, these problems can be amplified by cultural expectations that men be stoic. Men are told that they are not supposed to cry or show their emotions outwardly, that they are supposed to be self-reliant, to not ask for help, and that any illness, mental or physical, is a sign of weakness and a source of personal shame. A fundamental understanding of the similarities and differences in how males and females view, address and manage behavioral health issues is essential to providing care that is both clinically relevant and comfortable for patients. As society grapples with the serious issues of clinical depression and suicide, having a better understanding of these conditions within the framework of gender-based health care is appropriate.

Personal assessment

Is it hard for you to talk to your friends about emotional issues?

Background

The backdrop for any discussion about health and wellness for boys and men in the United States are the health disparities that exist. Despite significant advances in the recognition and treatment of medical conditions and the growing number of resources dedicated to health and wellness, men in America live shorter, less healthy lives than do American women. In addition, men die younger and at higher rates than women from nine of the ten leading causes of death in America (Men's Health Network, n.d.). In 2019, the Centers for Disease Control and Prevention [CDC] (2019) presented the very chilling statistic that there has been a significant decrease in life expectancy each year since 2015 among men, while life expectancy remained stable among women. This drop is, in part, due to the alarming rise in the suicide rate for boys and men.

Fundamental to understanding the issues involved in mental health for boys and men, it is necessary to have an appreciation of its potential root causes. The complexity of these root causes is underscored when you consider the integral role of cultural norms in forming ideas about appropriate behavior, expression and interpersonal interactions on a global level. Further, in heterogeneous societies, which commonly exist in major urban areas around the globe, the interplay of vastly different sociocultural overlays to normative behavior and emotional expression must be taken into account. In order to adequately understand the overall issues related to behavioral health and statistical reports of behavioral health issues, it is essential to understand the inherent factors that impact the reporting of mental health problems in boys and men. Many of these will be covered in more depth in later sections of this chapter, but at this juncture it should be noted that the differences in how females and males are acculturated to think about, communicate and act on physical health and wellness is magnified when it comes to behavioral health and wellness. Behavioral health issues can be found in schools, the workforce and the military, and they can have an adverse impact.

A global issue

Across the globe, mental health is an increasingly difficult and growing concern. Medical literature publications from around the world are replete with scientific, clinical and social scholarly articles that address these issues. A 2002 World Health Organization [WHO] report estimates that mental health issues contribute to 12.3% of all disability-adjusted life years, demonstrating a very significant impact on health status. Mental health issues may vary in type, etiology and co-morbidity from one society to another and from industrialized to non-industrialized countries, but they are, unfortunately, ubiquitous. In underdeveloped and developing countries, there are millions of people at risk of mental health problems unique to these locations due to, or complicated and worsened by, extreme poverty, war and social unrest, and significantly substandard overall living conditions, access to and quality of health care, poor nutrition, and quality of life circumstances.

The signs, symptoms, contributory and causative factors, and the diagnostic and treatment parameters for mental health matters differ along gender lines. WHO (2002) reports that in many industrialized countries men do not access health care services as regularly as women and frequently wait until late in a disease process to seek professional help. Men also have difficulty articulating emotional health issues. Globally, many men depend on the women in their lives for health care needs; as different social models of gender self-identification evolve, the social and clinical recognition and management of behavioral health issues must also evolve.

Expressing emotional hurt

The combination of genetics, evolution, acculturation, lack of emotionally expressive vocabulary, and the impact of stigma levied against weak boys and men all factor into how most males outwardly express emotional pain and behavioral health concerns in many countries around the world. These factors similarly also impact the way observers, including healthcare providers, receive and perceive social, behavioral, and even diagnostic clues given by men about behavioral health issues.

There is agreement in the literature (Salk, Hyde & Abramson, 2017; Tannenbaum, Greaves & Graham, 2016; Väänänen et al., 2014) that, in general, girls and women outwardly express emotional pain differently from boys and men. Boys and men will tend to withdraw and become more isolated and less communicative when under emotional stress than their female counterparts. In addition, they will begin to change their behavior and turn to things like excessive drinking, sexual excesses, spending hours gambling or on their computer (Legato, n.d.). These are all mechanisms to escape the pressures of their lives. External warning signs of severe emotional distress that may be at a critical stage may be a change in personality, a lot more irritability and even turning to violence. Girls and women are much more likely to reach out to people in their support network to ask for help when they are experiencing depression and to schedule appointments with their medical provider (Legato, n.d.). Their social support networks are generally more supportive and accepting of such dialogue. It should be noted that individual behaviors may vary.

Many who have depression are unaware of the underlying problems that triggered the condition, a situation that complicates both the expression and the treatment of the condition. Boys who act out feelings of depression, or other emotional hurt, are often labeled by family, teachers and clinicians who are untrained in dealing with behavioral health issues in males as angry, a loner, a nerd, quiet, withdrawn, or shy. Such mischaracterizations virtually ensure that boys and young men who are actually suffering from depression, anxiety, or some other mental or behavioral health issue will not receive medical treatment, and their symptoms and underlying conditions remain untreated. Because of the way some boys and men occasionally act out when depressed, anxious, or suffering from other behavioral health conditions, they are considered by society, and occasionally health care providers, as bad or dangerous.

Many boys and men do attempt to be open about their emotional challenges, but, in part because of their poor ability to express their emotions and in part because of acculturation, this frequently comes with societal obstacles. Even when boys and men develop the ability to express emotional pain, it is all too often viewed as weakness by those around them who are in the best position to help. Many boys and men who try to express their emotions frequently discover that there is no incentive in recognizing their problems, speaking up and trying to deal with them. The negative (or, at best, neutral) feedback they most frequently receive leads them to suffer in silence. In some, this leads to further issues such as isolation or antisocial behavior but in others it can lead to destructive behaviors toward themselves and/or others. Behavioral health concerns for males are made even more complex because all men are different. Sociocultural, socioeconomic, racial, educational and vocational issues, age, and a myriad of other factors play a large role in both the predisposition to and determinants of mental health in males.

Personal assessment

Do you think you have an adequate vocabulary to express emotional hurt? If no, why not?

Considerations in the community

One of the first places where behavioral health issues can, and should, be picked up is in the home and community. While there are numerous opportunities for family, friends, educators, community leaders, coaches and employers to help boys and men with emotional hurt there are many impediments. These include lack of awareness of the problem, no vocational training in recognition of problems, issues of privacy, lack of support, training and development of skills and, very importantly, a lack of skill, systems or guidance in triaging to needed next steps.

The existence and the nature of links between behavioral health issues and violence and other forms of criminal behavior is controversial (Fazel et al., 2015; Furukawa, 2015). Many male health experts are deeply concerned that because of sociological prejudice and fundamentally poor understanding of depression in males, at both the community and professional levels, all too many males are moved into the criminal justice system rather than into an active health care or community support environment. While this adversely impacts all boys and men, it has particularly extensive and devastating impact on those from dysfunctional living environments, low socio-economic circumstances and of ethnic and racial minorities (Riolo, Nguyen, Greden & King, 2005).

Suicide

The 2018 CDC report, *Suicide rates in the United States continue to increase* (Hedegaard, Curtin & Warner, 2018) sent shock waves through many parts of the mental health, health professions, and men's health advocacy communities because of its unprecedented findings. The report found an increase in U.S. suicides of more than 30% in half of the states since 1999, with a national-level model-estimated average annual percentage change for the overall suicide rate showing an increase of 1.5%. Suicide is only one, albeit the most serious, manifestation of depression or other mental health issues. Across all ages and ethnicities, American men die by suicide at far higher rates than women. According to the most recent CDC data, between the ages of 15 and 64, roughly 3.5 times more men than women die by suicide (2019). From 65 to 74, male suicides outnumber females by more than 4:1, for those over 74, the difference is a startling 9.3:1 (CDC, 2019). Overall, for males, suicide is the 7th leading cause of death, while for females, it's number 14 (CDC, 2019). Figure 8.1 shows the differences in male and female suicide rates in the U.S. since 2000. There are also differences in suicide rates by race in the United States. A CDC report (Stone et al., 2018) found that people in the U.S. who completed suicides were predominantly male (76.8%) and non-Hispanic white (83.6%), followed by African-American males (6.0%) and Hispanic males (5.4%).

Similar disparities in suicide rates by sex can be seen globally. According to WHO (2018), men die by suicide at a rate of 13.5 per 100,000; twice as high when compared to women at a rate of 7.7 per 100,000. In Europe, the rate of male suicide is significantly higher at 24.7 per 100,000 compared to females at 6.6 per 100,000 (WHO, 2018). Even in regions where suicide rates are lower than the world average, rates of suicide in males are still significantly higher than in females. For example, in the Eastern Mediterranean region, the average number of suicides is 3.9 per 100,000, while male rates are still high with a rate of 5.1 compared to 2.7 for females (WHO, 2018).

Personal assessment

Have you ever had a screening for behavioral health? If so, did you ask to be evaluated or did someone encourage you to do the assessment?

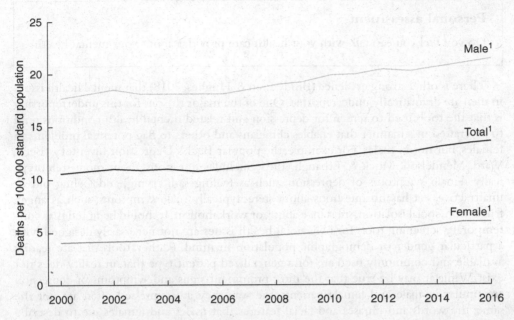

Figure 8.1 Age-adjusted suicide rates, by sex: United States, 2000–2016.

Notes:

1 Significant increasing trend from 2000 through 2016 with different rates of change over time, $p < 0.001$.

Suicides were identified using *International Classification of Diseases, 10th Revision*, underlying cause-of-death codes: U03, X60–X84, and Y87.0.

Age-adjusted death rates were calculated using the direct method and the 2000 standard population. Access data table for figure at www.cdc.gov/nchs/data/databriefs/db309_table.pdf#1

Source: Centers for Disease Control and Prevention (2019).

Male-specific screening tools

Many mental health professionals and clinicians cite that females are roughly twice as likely as males to be diagnosed with depression and other mental health issues (King, Horwitz, Czyz & Lindsay, 2017). However, others express concern that this number, while often quoted, does not convey the true magnitude of the problem and the true incidence of undiagnosed depression (Burton, 2012). This ratio represents the number of clinically diagnosed cases of depression, not the actual incidence. Because of the problems with self-reporting, lack of screening, lack of male-specific depression screening tools, willingness to treat and presentation of boys or men to be treated, most experts in men's health doubt that this represents the actual occurrence of depression in males. The 2:1 ratio may, in part, be a reflection of the fact that men present for medical encounters half as often as women do. And they're even less likely to seek help for mental health issues than physical health issues (King et al., 2017; Schrijvers, Bollen & Sabbe, 2012). Eliminating the 2:1 disparity in the number of visits could, theoretically, also eliminate the corresponding 2:1 difference in women's likelihood of being diagnosed with depression.

Personal assessment

Do you feel you can talk with your health care provider about your mental health?

There is other strong evidence (Brody, Pratt & Hughes, 2018) that mental health issues in men are dramatically underreported. One of the major reasons for this underreporting is that the tools used to screen for depression and related mental health conditions tend to be crafted in a manner that enables clinicians and others to flag potential problems in females, but not in males. For example, the popular Beck's Depression Inventory (Beck, Ward, Mendelson, Mock & Erbaugh, 1961) includes questions about more stereotypically female symptoms of depression, such as feeling sad, crying, and feeling old or unattractive, yet has no questions about stereotypically male symptoms, such as anger, frustration, social isolation, substance abuse, or workaholism. It should be noted that contemporary screening tools for behavioral health issues are not necessarily designed with a particular gender or demographic population in mind. Rather, tools that are readily available and commonly used are for a generalized patient type that, in reality, does not exist. While it may be true that the most prominent signs and symptoms of depression are similar in male and female patients, the way they are expressed often are not the same, the words and phrases and facial features that males and females use to describe emotional hurt are different (McDuff, Kodra, el Kaliouby & LaFrance, 2017) and their willingness to discuss their problems and the social acceptability of acknowledging them also differs.

Did you know?

Men's Health Network (2019) created a brief mental health screener for depression that was designed specifically with imagery, wording and relevance to males as a door knob hanger to be used in college dorms. Developing mental health screening tools that use verbiage, emotional cues and imagery pleasing to the different demographics of men is an important component of creating male-optimized screening tools.

Sleep and social media

For those who are anxious or depressed, social media, which includes apps such as Facebook, Snapchat and Instagram, may provide a way for men to reach out to others who are experiencing similar symptoms and find support online when they do not feel comfortable seeking support offline. Social media has allowed people to connect, not only with those around them, but with people around the world. While there has been some concern that spending a lot of time on social media can lead to depression, there has been no conclusive link between the use of social media and one's mental well-being (Best, Manktelow & Taylor, 2014; Jelenchick, Eickhoff & Moreno, 2013).

One of the negative impacts of using social media is dependent on when it's used, such as using it prior to bedtime, because of the blue light that is emitted from smartphones

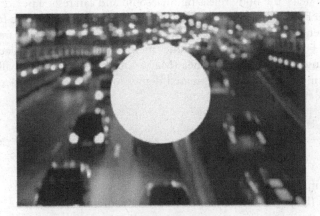

Recognize the Signs

■ Feeling sad, worthless, hopeless, or lonely
■ A drop in performance in school or on the job
■ Feeling angry, irritable, tense, or on edge
■ Withdrawing from family and friends
■ Loss of interest in your favorite activities
■ Feelings of guilt for no apparent reason
■ Change in sleeping patterns
■ Unexplained weight loss or gain
■ Loss of self-confidence
■ Difficulty making decisions or concentrating
■ Difficulty completing simple daily tasks
■ Thoughts of death or suicide
■ Feeling like your whole life is coming apart

You Can Take Control!

If you or a friend experience any of the above symptoms for more than two weeks, or if any of these are interfering with your life, go to a wellness center, or talk to a counselor, your pastor or a trusted friend right away.

Not getting the help you need could only make the problem worse.

Help & Resources

National Suicide Prevention Lifeline
800-273-TALK (8255)
www.suicidepreventionlifeline.org

Substance Abuse & Mental Health Services Administration
877-SAMHSA-7 (726-4247)
www.samhsa.gov

ULifeline: Online Resource for Students
www.ulifeline.org

Your Head: An Owner's Manual
www.blueprintformenshealth.com

Figure 8.2 Example of a screening tool created specifically for men.
Source: By permission of the *Men's Health Network* (2019) © www.Menshealthnetwork.org.

and tablets. This blue light can delay the body releasing melatonin and can reset a person's internal clock (National Sleep Foundation, n.d.-a). This can be especially problematic for men, since they rebound slower when they experience sleep deprivation, when compared to women (National Sleep Foundation, n.d.-b). Some men may already face sleep challenges, as they are more susceptible to sleep apnea (Mayo Clinic, 2018). Additionally, general life stress and attempting to cope with untreated depression can also make sleep difficult for men (National Sleep Foundation, n.d.-c).

Learn more

him + *his* is a collection of images and written contributions from over 100 authors on men and mental health (Kleih, 2018). Learn more at www.antennebooks.com/product/him-his/.

The role of stigma

Another major obstacle to recognizing, diagnosing and treating mental health issues in men is stigma. The 2000 U.S. Surgeon General's Report (Satcher, 2000) addresses the issue of stigma and its role in advancing the care of people with behavioral health conditions. In the report, Dr. Satcher notes that of those who have a severe mental illness, almost half will not seek treatment, often because of the stigma that is associated with mental illness in the United States.

The way stigma is perceived, reacted to, and dealt with is very different for men and women. Some men are not even aware that their reactions or aversion to dealing with depression or other behavioral health issues are the result of their concern about stigma, and thus don't even identify with the term. The way men interact with other men is also different from the way women interact with other women. As a result, even the coping mechanisms boys and men may develop to deal with perceived feelings of stigma are different. Women tend to react verbally and emotionally, while men react in a physical way. This can be manifested in a number of behavioral traits such as anger, substance abuse or by withdrawing. The underpinnings of how men and boys react to and deal with emotional hurt and issues begins at a very young age. One of the first things a boy hears when he injures himself as a youngster is that when he talks about it he quickly gets shut down with a phrase or reaction that telegraphs *Big boys don't cry*, *Play through it*, or *Man up!* One of the consequences of this type of response from loved ones is that boys often feel that reacting to physical hurt is a bad thing and this, more often than not, later on translates into an aversion to reacting to emotional hurt. Overall, parents speak more to infant girls than to infant boys (Lovas, 2011; O'Brien & Nagle, 1987). But, the content of that speech is even more important than the volume. Researchers have documented this in a recent study that found that both mothers and fathers use more words describing emotions with 4-year-old girls than with boys the same age (Aznar & Tenenbaum, 2016).

In his own words

Anonymous

I get frustrated when I'm emotional. It can be crippling, because I can't do other things when I feel it. It's really tough to be consistently strong and composed in front of everyone when there's stuff being thrown at me, and I don't know how to deal with it. I'm a very emotional person, and I don't hide it. Another thing of 'masculinity' is holding all those things back. Which I don't think is a good idea, because that makes it so much worse.

(*Source*: personal communication from Kayla Hense, 2019)

Urging boys to suppress and even ignore their emotions starts long before children are even able to play. Several studies have found that mothers and fathers both tend to speak more to infant girls than to infant boys, cuddle infant boys less than they do girls, and respond more quickly to an infant girl's cries than to a crying boy's. Similarly, we perceive the identical behavior differently, depending on whether we think we're watching a boy or a girl. In one fascinating experiment, Condry and Condry (1976) showed a group of people a film of a 9-month-old child playing with a jack in the box and were asked to describe the child's reaction when the jack popped. Half of the viewers were told they were watching a girl, the other half saw the same film but were told they were watching a boy. Those in the boy group said that the child was angry when the jack popped. Those in the girl group said the child was frightened. Most of us would respond very differently to a frightened child than to an angry one.

A direct and dire result of stigma is the impact it has on boys and men of color with behavioral health conditions. The degree to which stigma impacts these communities and individuals cannot be overstated. According to a recent report from the CDC, between 1999 and 2017, the overall suicide rate for Native Americans increased substantially (Curtin & Hedegaard, 2019). However, for Native American males, the jump in age-adjusted suicide rates was even more startling, rising from 19.8 per 100,000 to 33.8 per 100,000 population, a 71% increase (Curtin & Hedegaard, 2019). African-American and other boys and men of color in particular are, from a young age, vigorously told by parents, community influencers and peers to *keep your feelings to yourself* because of the fear of parents and older peers that expressions of feelings might fuel hostile racial stereotypes. In many communities of color, stigma against weakness or any semblance of mental health issues is very pronounced.

The prevalence of behavioral health conditions and the lack of recognition and care in African-American and Latino boys and men is shockingly high. Men of color are less likely to receive the mental health care they need when compared to white men (PBS, n.d.). They may face many barriers because of their race, including prejudice, poverty and a lack of access to services (PBS, n.d.). An additional barrier is the lack of cultural competence on the part of healthcare workers. Many experts feel that it is important to develop and nurture emotional first aid programs and community-based training programs that encompass gender-specific techniques and sensitivities to directly and early on address problems. By working with churches and local community groups, men can work to reduce the stigma and other barriers that exist and increase the support for more culturally specific initiatives.

Post-traumatic stress disorder

In older individuals, particularly men who are engaged in work that involves immersion in dangerous, traumatic and life-threatening activities, such as military, first-responders and law enforcement, post-traumatic stress disorder (PTSD) can manifest in subtle and sometimes not-so-subtle ways. Typically, PTSD creates difficult socialization issues, but occasionally, it results in violent behavior. There are numerous other examples of male loners who have emotional pain—never recognized, disclosed, or identified in a medical encounter—that at some point manifests as violent rage. According to the Anxiety and Depression Association of America (ADAA, 2015), PTSD can also be found in younger men and, occasionally in boys. This is particularly the case when there are significantly stressful, impaired or abusive relationships with parents, siblings, peers, other caregivers, such as uncles or aunts, or because of difficult or traumatic environments in school or day care settings (ADAA, 2015).

The symptoms and diagnosis of PTSD are complex and dependent on multiple variables, but there are common symptoms. One of the symptoms is re-experiencing the trauma. This might occur through nightmares and flashbacks (ADAA, n.d.). Choosing to avoid people and places that remind people of the original trauma, in addition to finding it hard to sleep, getting angry quickly and finding it hard to concentrate, are other common symptoms.

Learn more

Your Head: An Owner's Manual is a book about men and mental health, covering topics such as depression, anxiety disorders, stress and PTSD (Brott & Men's Health Network Advisory Board, 2008). Learn more at www.menshealthnetwork.org/library/ownersmanual.pdf.

Moving forward

There is much work in both the scientific and general community needed to address the issues of mental health in boys and men. In 2015, the United Nations General Assembly announced that both substance abuse and mental health would be included in the Sustainable Development Goals. While this is a huge step forward for topics that have been too often stigmatized, it's important to note that how this is addressed globally will differ based on the local population. From countries such as Sierra Leone, which is still dealing with the trauma of a decade-long civil war, to countries like Liberia that only has one psychiatric hospital (Gberie, 2017), each country will need to identify strategies to promote positive mental health.

Many U.S. colleges and universities, as well as some primary and secondary schools, have put programs in place to support staff in understanding, recognizing and assisting students with such problems, as well as for students at risk of such problems. It is difficult to know just what percentage of educational institutions have programs, but the overall consensus is that the number is growing as recognition of the problem is growing. One novel approach is the use of an online virtual system called Kognito on many college campuses. Kognito

(2019) is designed to help students begin a dialogue about emotional distress. For student athletes in the United States, there are unique amounts of stress because of the combined demands of academics and athletics. The National Collegiate Athletic Association (NCAA, n.d.) has developed a program model to help athletic staff and other support personnel on campus help student athletes deal with mental health issues that may develop.

What needs more attention is how to meet the needs of men who aren't enrolled in school. How these needs are addressed will need to be tailored to the specific population they are trying to target, which may differ depending on their location (urban vs. suburban vs. rural), age and race. For example, for men of color, there need to be efforts to increase community outreach, so that these men have safe spaces of entry as a way of accessing mental health, instead of being forced to seek care by friends and family, or being introduced to care through the criminal justice system. These types of services are being offered in certain parts of the United Kingdom for African and Caribbean men (Keating, 2007).

As a response to the rise in male suicide, the Men's Health Network established priorities to form the elements of a platform to move forward. These include the creation of male-specific screening tools for behavioral health conditions and developing education and training for clinicians and the community that focus on helping people communicate with males about behavioral health issues (Giorgianni Jr, & Brott, 2019). Other priorities include creating legislation that helps to support the well-being of males across the lifespan, as well as creating a single resource center that would store and disseminate information about best practices and information about policies that focus on male health (Giorgianni Jr. & Brott, 2019).

While efforts are being made to identify what needs to be done to help men and boys address mental health, a concern is that it's not happening fast enough. Not only does it appear that the mental health problems that plague males in our society aren't getting any better, they may in fact be getting worse. A 2019 report by Blue-Cross Blue-Shield found that, in general, Millennials (those born between 1981 and 1996) were only living at about 95% of their projected optimal health. A 2018 report found that 30% of Millennials self-reported feeling lonely and are more likely than older generations to report that they have no acquaintances (25%), no friends (22%), no close friends (27%), and no best friends (30%) (Ballard, 2019). These findings show a dramatic difference when compared to prior generations. The links between feelings of social isolation, lack of emotional lexicon, poor health care focus and depression and related behavioral health issues is an important one in this generation, and generations to come.

References

Anxiety and Depression Association of America. (n.d.). *Symptoms of PTSD*. Retrieved from https://adaa.org/understanding-anxiety/posttraumatic-stress-disorder-ptsd/symptoms

Anxiety and Depression Association of America. (2015). *PTSD symptoms in children age six and younger*. Retrieved from https://adaa.org/living-with-anxiety/children/posttraumatic-stress-disorder-ptsd/symptoms

Aznar, A., & Tenenbaum, H. R. (2016). Parent–child positive touch: Gender, age, and task differences. *Journal of Nonverbal Behavior*, 40(4), 317–333.

Ballard, J. (2019). Millennials are the loneliest generation. *YouGov*. Retrieved from https://today.yougov.com/topics/lifestyle/articles-reports/2019/07/30/loneliness-friendship-new-friends-poll-survey

Beck, A. T., Ward, C. H., Mendelson, M., Mock, J., & Erbaugh, J. (1961). An inventory for measuring depression. *Archives of General Psychiatry, 4*(6), 561–571.

Best, P., Manktelow, R., & Taylor, B. (2014). Online communication, social media and adolescent wellbeing: A systematic narrative review. *Children and Youth Services Review, 41*, 27–36.

BlueCross BlueShield. (2019). *The health of millennials.* Retrieved from https://www.bcbs.com/the-health-of-america/reports/the-health-of-millennials

Brody, D. J., Pratt, L. A., & Hughes, J. P. (2018). Prevalence of depression among adults aged 20 and over: United States, 2013–2016. *NCHS Data Brief,* (303), 1–8.

Brott, A., & Men's Health Network Advisory Board. (2008). *Your Head: An owner's manual.* Washington, DC: Men's Health Network.

Burton, N. (2012). The 7 reasons why depression is more common in women. *Psychology Today.* Retrieved from www.psychologytoday.com/blog/hide-andseek/201205/the-7-reasons-why-depression-is-morecommon-in-women.

Centers for Disease Control and Prevention. (2019). *At-a-glance table.* Retrieved from www.cdc.gov/nchs/hus/ataglance.htm

Condry, J., & Condry, S. (1976). Sex differences: A study of the eye of the beholder. *Child Development,* 812–819.

Curtin, S. C., & Hedegaard, H. (2019). Suicide rates for females and males by race and ethnicity: United States, 1999 and 2017. *NCHS Health E-Stat.* 2019.

Fazel, S., Wolf, A., Chang, Z., Larsson, H., Goodwin, G. M., & Lichtenstein, P. (2015). Depression and violence: A Swedish population study. *The Lancet Psychiatry, 2*(3), 224–232.

Furukawa, T. A. (2015). The relationship between depression and violent crime. *The Lancet Psychiatry, 2*(3), 193–194.

Gberie, L. (2017). Mental illness: Invisible but devastating. *Africa Renewal.* Retrieved from www.un.org/africarenewal/magazine/december-2016-march-2017/mental-illness-invisible-devastating

Giorgianni Jr., S. J., & Brott, A. (2019). Conference summary: Behavioral health aspects of depression and anxiety in the American male. *Men's Health Network.* Retrieved from www.menshealthnetwork.org/library/depression-anxiety-males-report.pdf

Hedegaard, H., Curtin, S. C., & Warner, M. (2018). *Suicide rates in the United States continue to increase.* US Department of Health and Human Services, Centers for Disease Control and Prevention, National Center for Health Statistics.

Jelenchick, L. A., Eickhoff, J. C., & Moreno, M. A. (2013). "Facebook depression?" Social networking site use and depression in older adolescents. *Journal of Adolescent Health, 52*(1), 128–130.

Keating, F. (2007). African and Caribbean men and mental health. *Race Equity Foundation.* Retrieved from https://raceequalityfoundation.org.uk/wp-content/uploads/2018/03/health-brief5.pdf

King, C. A., Horwitz, A., Czyz, E., & Lindsay, R. (2017). Suicide risk screening in healthcare settings: Identifying males and females at risk. *Journal of Clinical Psychology in Medical Settings, 24*(1), 8–20.

Kleih, H. S. (2018). *him + his.* London: Antenne Books.

Legato, M. (n.d.). *Women and men, how do they respond differently to stress?* Retrieved from www.empowher.com/emotional-health/content/women-and-men-how-do-they-respond-differently-stress-dr-legato-video

Lovas, G. S. (2011). Gender and patterns of language development in mother-toddler and father-toddler dyads. *First Language, 31*(1), 83–108.

Mayo Clinic. (2018). *Sleep apnea.* Retrieved from www.mayoclinic.org/diseases-conditions/sleep-apnea/symptoms-causes/syc-2037763

McDuff, D., Kodra, E., el Kaliouby, R., & LaFrance, M. (2017). A large-scale analysis of sex differences in facial expressions. *PloS One, 12*(4), e0173942.

Men's Health Network. (n.d). *Top causes of death by race, sex, and ethnicity–2016.* Retrieved from www.menshealthnetwork.org/library/causesofdeath.pdf

Men's Health Network. (2019). *Door hangers: don't race thru life feeling blue.* Retrieved from www.mhnshop.shoppingcartsplus.com/catalog/item/361339/8706226.htm

National Sleep Foundation. (n.d.-a). *How blue light affects kids & sleep.* Retrieved from www. sleepfoundation.org/articles/how-blue-light-affects-kids-sleep

National Sleep Foundation. (n.d.-b). *How does a man's sleep differ from a woman's?* Retrieved from www.sleep.org/articles/man-vs-woman-sleep/

National Sleep Foundation. (n.d.-c). *Unique sleep issues men face.* Retrieved from https://www.sleep. org/articles/unique-sleep-issues-men/

NCAA. (n.d.). *Developing and evaluating a model program for supporting the mental health of student athletes.* Retrieved from www.ncaa.org/about/resources/research/developing-and-evaluating-model-program-supporting-mental-health-student-athletes.

O'Brien, M., & Nagle, K. J. (1987). Parents' speech to toddlers: The effect of play context. *Journal of Child Language, 14*(2), 269–279.

PBS. (n.d.). *Depression. Out of the shadows. Depression in communities of color.* Retrieved from www-tc.pbs.org/wgbh/takeonestep/depression/pdf/dep_color.pdf

Riolo, S. A., Nguyen, T. A., Greden, J. F., & King, C. A. (2005). Prevalence of depression by race/ethnicity: Findings from the National Health and Nutrition Examination Survey III. *American Journal of Public Health, 95*(6), 998–1000.

Salk, R. H., Hyde, J. S., & Abramson, L. Y. (2017). Gender differences in depression in representative national samples: Meta-analyses of diagnoses and symptoms. *Psychological Bulletin, 143*(8), 783.

Satcher, D. (2000). Mental health: A report of the Surgeon General—Executive summary. *Professional Psychology: Research and Practice, 31*(1), 5.

Schrijvers, D. L., Bollen, J., & Sabbe, B. G. (2012). The gender paradox in suicidal behavior and its impact on the suicidal process. *Journal of Affective Disorders, 138*(1–2), 19–26.

Stone, D. M., Simon, T. R., Fowler, K. A., Kegler, S. R., Yuan, K., Holland, K. M., … & Crosby, A. E. (2018). Vital signs: Trends in state suicide rates—United States, 1999–2016 and circumstances contributing to suicide—27 states, 2015. *Morbidity and Mortality Weekly Report, 67*(22), 617.

Tannenbaum, C., Greaves, L., & Graham, I. D. (2016). Why sex and gender matter in implementation research. *BMC Medical Research Methodology, 16*(1), 145.

Väänänen, J. M., Isomaa, R., Kaltiala-Heino, R., Fröjd, S., Helminen, M., & Marttunen, M. (2014). Decrease in self-esteem mediates the association between symptoms of social phobia and depression in middle adolescence in a sex-specific manner: a 2-year follow-up of a prospective population cohort study. *BMC Psychiatry, 14*(1), 79.

World Health Organization. (n.d.). *Mental health included in the UN Sustainable Development Goals.* Retrieved from www.who.int/mental_health/SDGs/en/

World Health Organization. (2002). *Gender and mental health.* Retrieved from www.who.int/gender/other_health/genderMH.pdf

World Health Organization. (2018). *Suicide.* Retrieved from http://apps.who.int/gho/data/node. sdg.3-4-viz-2?lang=en

9 Healthy relationships

Barry Sharp

From the early days of history, men have been in relationships and not always successfully. According to Judeo-Christian theology, mankind began in the Garden of Eden where Adam and Eve were created by God to be in a relationship with each other and with their creator. This was short lived as they were kicked out of Eden for eating the forbidden fruit (Common English Bible, 2011). Not only did their actions separate them from being with their creator in the garden, but Adam dishonored Eve when he justified his actions by putting the blame on Eve for giving him the fruit, setting a precedent that men have repeated ever since.

While this story is from a religious perspective, and it's not the only story of how men and women came to be on this earth, it is reflective of men in relationships. Look around and watch men and their relationships – personal, professional and community. All men have had times when their relationships are wonderful and times when they are not. Relationships require work and dedication, talking and listening, give and take and occasionally repentance and forgiveness.

Popular culture likes to picture men as rugged, individualistic, border-line loners who don't need others in their life, or as the Alpha male who is constantly driven to be on top, whether it's the corporate ladder or political office, and will do whatever it takes to be there including using peer pressure to force others to do things they might not otherwise choose to do. The reality is that men are healthier and more successful when they are in healthy relationships with others.

However, healthy relationships don't just happen. While the elements of a healthy relationship are discussed in more detail in this chapter, the foundations for having a healthy relationship are poured as a boy learns how men treat others in friendships, intimate and professional relationships. Are others treated respectfully with their needs taking a higher priority than one's own needs? Are others pressured to do things they would not normally choose to do? As a man, one needs to be aware of how they interact with others and the impact those actions have. In the era of the #MeToo movement, women are rightly standing up against men's inappropriate behaviors that might have been considered as the norm or "boys being boys" a generation or two ago. Men are being held to a higher standard than years ago, but a standard in which all individuals are treated with respect and value.

Research on the impact of relationships on health has traditionally focused on married versus unmarried adults. According to the Centers for Disease Control and Prevention (CDC) those studies have found that married people are generally healthier than unmarried persons (Schoenborn, 2004). Unmarried persons include those who have never married and those who are divorced, separated or widowed. In their research, two main concepts emerged to explain this finding – marriage protection and marriage selection (Schoenborn, 2004). Marriage protection suggests that married people have more advantages in terms of economic resources, social and psychological support, and support for a healthy lifestyle. Marriage selection refers to the idea that healthier people get married and stay married, whereas less healthy people do not marry or are more likely to become separated, divorced or widowed. Other studies have also shown that marriage is associated with longer longevity and that never being married was the strongest predictor of premature mortality (Kaplan & Kronick, 2006).

These overall findings have remained consistent despite the changes in society that have redefined the meaning of being married since this research began more than a half century ago. These changes have included seeing the age of first marriage increasing; divorce, once considered taboo, is now commonplace; living with a domestic partner outside of a legal union as well as the legalization of marriage between same-sex partners; and the changing dynamics and definition of what constitutes a family unit or household.

In this chapter, readers will gain an understanding of:

- what a healthy relationship looks like;
- the types of relationships and roles men play in relationships;
- the health impacts that come from being in a relationship.

Personal assessment

As you read this chapter, reflect on your own relationships with others, particularly intimate relationships. Are those relationships healthy? Does your behavior – actions and words – show respect and compassion for the other person in the relationship? Will the actions you do today be something you will be proud of in 30 years or are they something you hope will be forgotten by everyone involved? Would you be comfortable if your family learned what you did from a news report?

Healthy relationships

Boys learn to be men, in part, by watching men who came before. Working to fit in with the expectations learned from watching others creates a peer pressure to behave a certain way and/or believe a certain way, in order to be accepted by the group. Often this is associated with negative health behaviors or taking risky actions that could result in a negative outcome. It is also used in marketing to make you think you need to purchase something in order to be considered cool, hip or sophisticated.

In relationships, peer pressure can set the tone for what behavior is expected as it relates to dress, activities, and can be as innocent as trying a new food while on a date or as sinister as forcing someone to participate in unwanted sexual behaviors. At the workplace, it can influence an unwritten dress code for what is acceptable and considered professional dress and where the group goes out to lunch on Tuesdays. Likewise, in a community, peer pressure helps to maintain the community standards for what behaviors are and are not acceptable, including how men treat women.

The ability to use peer pressure to reduce or re-enforce behaviors related to sexual aggression against women was also studied and researchers found that men's discussions with men about women can foster an environment that encourages or discourages sexual violence (Jacques-Tiura et al., 2015). Men who were in groups that consistently used language that objectified women perceived more peer pressure to have sex by any means – including intoxication or by force – and were more uncomfortable with egalitarian (positive and uplifting) statements (Jacques-Tiura et al., 2015). Men who used more egalitarian language to describe women and their relationship to women felt less pressure to have sex (Jacques-Tiura et al., 2015). By simply setting the example of treating women (and all others) with respect and as peers, men can influence their own behavior and the behavior of others, which can lead to healthy relationships.

Longtime relationship researcher John Gottman and his team focused their work looking at married couples whose relationships were in trouble, finding those common elements which could predict a marriage that was heading toward divorce with a 90% accuracy (Gottman & Levenson, 1999, 2002). Those common elements were called The Four Horsemen by Gottman and his colleagues as a reference to their being almost apocalyptic in ending a marriage. In describing these elements, they also listed the antidotes to these actions as ways individuals can strengthen relationships. The Four Horsemen are:

- *Criticism*: verbally attacking the other partner's personality or character. The antidote is to use gentler language to approach the issue by talking about feelings and using "I" statements to describe those feelings and expressing a positive need.
- *Contempt*: attacking sense of self with an intent to insult or abuse. To avoid sounding contemptuous, build a culture of appreciation by reminding yourself of your partner's positive qualities and find gratitude for any positive actions taken.
- *Defensiveness*: victimizing yourself to ward off a perceived attack and reverse the blame. The opposite action would be to take responsibility for your actions, accept your partner's perspective on issues and offer an apology for any wrongdoing on your part.
- *Stonewalling*: withdrawing to avoid conflict and convey disapproval, distance and separation. To avoid stonewalling, do physiological self-soothing by taking a break (a time-out) and spend that time doing something soothing and distracting so that you can come back to the issue with a refreshed attitude.

Gottman and Levenson (2002) identified that relationships were most at risk for divorce in the first seven years of marriage (when more than half of all divorces occur) and the second is in midlife when couples may have young teenagers at home. The first period is characterized by a relationship that is volatile and highly emotional (Gottman & Levenson, 2002). The second period is what may be seen as the lowest point in marital satisfaction as this period has high external demands on the relationship (work/career, children's activities, ageing parents and finances) leaving little time and resources to focus on the relationship itself (Gottman & Levenson, 2002).

Gottman and Levenson (2002) found that couples who stay together displayed a positive affect to each other, often using humor as a means to lighten the gravity of the discussion over issues, as well as the ability for men to take advice and counsel from their wives. Likewise, researchers found that in same-sex relationships, couples are more upbeat in the face of conflict and use more affection and humor when bringing up difficult conversations when compared to straight couples (Gottman et al., 2003).

Researchers speculate that part of the reason is that in same-sex relationships equality between the partners is highly valued, while in heterosexual relationships partners are faced with the standard status hierarchy between men and women (Gottman et al., 2003). This status hierarchy can lead to hostility, particularly from women who have less power, and who typically are more aware of and bring up issues with the relationship (Gottman et al., 2003).

Did you know?

The Gottman Institute (2019) website offers information for couples, parents and professionals on healthy relationships. To learn more, visit www.gottman.com/.

To understand what makes a healthy relationship, one needs to know how to identify the signs of an unhealthy relationship as well as a healthy relationship. The University of Washington (Health Promotion Staff, 2014) created a website that clearly defines healthy and unhealthy activities within a relationship. An unhealthy relationship is characterized by behaviors that frequently occur that cause stress and pressure and signifies that one person is trying to, or is in a position to, exert power or pressure on the other person. This can be exhibited in manipulation to change behaviors, appearance or pressure to engage in unwanted sexual activities (see Table 9.1). Healthy relationships, on the other hand, are based on mutual respect, caring and compassion and add value to those involved in the relationship. While no relationship is perfect, and even in long-term relationships there are ups and downs, overall, a healthy relationship will bring joy and happiness to those in the relationship and allow for each to grow as individuals and as a couple, group or community.

Things that make a relationship healthy will include mutual respect, trust, honesty, support for each other, a fairness or equality in the give and take within the relationship, maintaining separate identities and maintaining a sense of playfulness and fondness for each other. Many couples report that being able to laugh with each other is an important

Table 9.1 A comparison of signs of healthy and unhealthy relationships

Signs of a healthy relationship	Signs of an unhealthy relationship
Taking care of yourself and having good self-esteem independent of the relationship	Putting one person before the other to the point of neglecting yourself or your partner
Being able to express thoughts, feelings and fears without fear of consequences	Worrying about the reaction of the other person during a disagreement
Having respect for sexual boundaries	Feeling obligated or forced to have sex
Trusting each other and being honest with each other	Lacking privacy or being forced to share everything with the other person
Feeling secure and comfortable	Having to justify actions, such as where you go or who you see
Maintaining and respecting each other's individuality	Feeling pressure to change (values, activities, appearance) for the other person or changing the other person to suit your desires

Source: Adapted from the website http://depts.washington.edu/hhpccweb/health-resource/healthy-vs-unhealthy-relationships/.

element in a long-term relationship. This does not happen magically or overnight. Building a healthy relationship takes time and commitment to both the relationship and to the shared goals of those in the relationship.

Relationships are full of give and take, shared thoughts, shared goals and putting the other person's needs ahead of your own. Each person will influence the other by either helping them consider new points of view or reinforcing beliefs and behaviors, as was suggested when discussing peer pressure. Being in a healthy relationship allows for this to happen and encourages positive influences in building the relationship's identity, beliefs and values.

Learn more

The Buddy System: Understanding male friendships (Greif, 2008) explores male relationships based on 400 interviews with men to reveal the dynamics of male friendships.

Types and roles of relationships

While most of the research on men's relationships focuses on intimate relationships, men function in a world where there are a variety of differing relationships that individuals move in and out of during the course of a day, week or lifespan from the personal one-on-one relationship to relationships with community. Depending on the relationship with those around them, the role played may be different. To clarify for discussion, here are some general definitions for these various types of relationships:

- *Personal*: These are relationships with those with whom we are closest, such as a spouse or significant other (intimate or marital relationship) or a parent or sibling (familial relationship). Friends also fall under personal relationships, but the level of closeness in the relationship can vary from very intimate friends, i.e. best friends or BFF friends, who you see often and constantly do activities with, to acquaintances who you know as friends but do not have a level of intimacy, such as a neighbor.
- *Professional*: These are the relationships that occur while at work and can include those we work with, work for, and/or are supervised by. This can include co-workers, customers, contractors, consultants or any other person with whom an individual comes into contact during working hours.
- *Community*: These are relationships where you are part of a larger community or organization and the relationships are not one-on-one, but rather one-on-many, and the focus isn't on the individual but on the group outcome or benefit to others. Examples of this can include membership in volunteer organizations, such as a civic club, a volunteer fire department or volunteering at a school; being involved in government or schools; or participating or membership in a religious organization.

Research has shown that social connectedness has a direct relation to health (Ashida & Heaney, 2008). People who are involved with friends, social organizations and volunteering have less illness, fewer mental health issues, greater longevity and have better economic outcomes than those who don't. Researchers at Carnegie Mellon University found that those with more diverse social networks even have fewer colds (Cohen, Brissette, Skoner

& Doyle, 2000). And those who do not have social support can cut their risks of dying in the next year in half by joining a group. For men who see themselves as independents who do not see a reason for social support, this mindset can cause increased health problems and a shorter lifespan.

To fully understand and embrace a man's role in creating social support, it is necessary to understand how men can, and do, function in relationships with other men (McKenzie, Collings, Jenkin & River, 2018). Researchers examined men's support networks, help-seeking behaviors and health-promoting practices, as well as collected information through interviews, and found that men have four key patterns of practice as it relates to the relationships (McKenzie et al., 2018). Summaries of the four patterns identified by McKenzie et al. (2018) are listed below:

- *Compartmentalizing*: Men see social relationships with men as being primarily based on shared social or physical activities with little talk about personal issues. Women, however, are more intimate and confiding, sharing personal information more freely with other women. Ironically, men also feel more comfortable in sharing their personal feelings with women – men share activities with men and get their emotional support from women. The downside of compartmentalizing is that the relationships with other men are activity based and prone to wane when the time demands of family or work increase – leaving few opportunities for socializing with friends or pursuing his own interests. It may also cause men to overly rely on women (such as their spouse) for emotional support.

- *Difficulties in confiding*: Some men do try to confide their feelings only to be met with feelings of inadequacy in that either their words do not truly convey their feelings or that the male friend in whom they are confiding doesn't want to participate in that level of emotional sharing, thus creating an uncomfortable setting for both. Part of this is that because men don't share as often or as deeply as women do with other women, they have not developed the skills to find the right words to share their feelings, and men have not developed the skills to simply listen empathetically without trying to solve the problem. This difficulty then leads men back to confiding with women to get needed emotional support.

- *An independent guy*: Men who describe themselves as self-sufficient and who do not need an emotional or social relationship. They may have networks of family and friends available, but they do not use them for fear of damaging their independent persona. This can result in men having to maintain a façade of control and success when the reality is that they are struggling to deal with the issues in their life, thus creating an almost superficial relationship based on shared activities and interests without the deep emotional connection. This can be dangerous when the issues in life become overwhelming or public, or the persona and/or relationships are not strong enough to provide the support needed to heal and rebuild.

- *Reaching out*: These are men who have developed close relationships with other men that are based on self-disclosure and openness about their private lives and feelings. This usually occurs when men have significant events in their lives that created the opportunity for emotional bonding, such as shared military experiences or serious health issues. In these male relationships, the friendships are deep and lasting and are focused on more than shared activities or interests, but concern for the other person's well-being and the ability to ask questions to draw out answers that helped each other to process their feelings to allow healing and improved mental health.

As can be expected, each of these relationship roles will impact an individual's capacity for developing the social support necessary to have relationships at the individual, professional and community levels. Being a person who compartmentalizes would have limited effect on their ability to be successful in the professional or community worlds, and it would impact their ability to create personal relationships at the individual level. An independent mindset might prevent someone from becoming active in community activities unless they see a personal benefit. An individual who is interested in reaching out may have limited success in the professional and community networks where success is measured in meeting the goals of the organization rather than the creation of individual relationships. That said, all organizations are built on the relationships that those involved have with each other, so it is important to build those networks in order that information can be shared, activities completed and goals met.

Health impacts

A study from Austria specifically looked at the impact of being in community with others to examine the health effects of those 50 years of age and older and found that both community conflict and community connectedness are related to an individual's health (Bowen & Luy, 2016). High levels of community conflicts were associated with participants reporting worse health, independent of the individual's own involvement in the conflict (Bowen & Luy, 2016). Conversely, those who reported being more connected to their communities reported better health (Bowen & Luy, 2016).

Schoenborn (2004) reported that being in a relationship had the biggest impact on men in the 18–44 and 45–64 age ranges, and the impact was bigger on men than women. Except for overweight or obesity, men reported being healthier than women and overall married men were healthier than other men (Schoenborn, 2004). Specifically, men who were living with a partner did not show as great a health benefit as those men who were married and those who were divorced reported being the unhealthiest (Schoenborn, 2004). It's important to note that for this research, marital status is defined by the respondent and may not be representative of a traditional, legal marriage status or if the other spouse was living in the home at the time of the survey. Those surveyed chose the category they felt best identified their situation.

Data from the U.S. Longitudinal Study of Aging, 1984–1990 (Goldman, Korenman & Weinstein, 1995) showed that marital status impacts even the oldest, with widowed men being at a higher risk of being disabled than married men. However, while unmarried men had variations in health, widowed persons had poorer health (Goldman, Korenman, & Weinstein, 1995). But divorced or single individuals didn't have that same outcome (Ramezankhani, Azizi & Hadaegh, 2019). In comparison, a study among couples aged 18, 21 and 24 years, who were followed for seven years, found that married couples had higher levels of well-being than single individuals and that men (but not women) reported less depression, and women (but not men) reported fewer alcohol problems (Horwitz, White & Howell-White, 1996).

A British study of data collected in the British Regional Health Study (Ebrahim, Wannamethee, McCallum, Walker, & Shaper, 1995) found similar results. The study of 7,735 men aged 40–59 from 1978 to 1980 showed that men who had never married had an increased risk of cardiovascular disease mortality and noncancer, non-cardiovascular mortality (Ebrahim et al., 1995). This increased risk was after adjustment for potentially confounding variables such as age, social class, smoking, history of cardiovascular disease or diabetes mellitus, hypertension medications, weight, physical activity, alcohol use or employment status. Divorced or separated men were not at risk of mortality and widowed men were only at increased risk of non-cardiovascular mortality causes (Ebrahim et al., 1995). Interestingly, men who divorced during the study period were at increased risk for both cardiovascular diseases and other non-cardiovascular disease mortality (Ebrahim et al., 1995). This increase in risk was not seen in men who became widowed. While their study did not find conclusive reasoning for the differences, the researchers did suggest that it was possible that the social support offered by marriage exerts a protective effect for some men (Ebrahim et al., 1995).

Likewise, a population-based study of men and women in Japan found a significant increase in cardiovascular and all-cause mortality in men who had never married when compared to a married group (Schultz et al., 2017). Similar findings were observed in a study in Iran which found that being single in men was associated with a 55% increased risk of hypertension, even after adjusting for traditional risk factors, and that never-married men had a 2.17 times higher all-cause mortality risk when compared to married men (Ramezankhani et al., 2019).

While the research showing that men in relationships have better outcomes than men who aren't married is overwhelming, research also shows that men in relationships where the spouse has chronic health conditions increases the risk for both spouses to suffer from the same conditions (Stimpson & Peek, 2005). A wife with a medical history of hypertension, diabetes, arthritis and cancer was associated with higher odds that the husband would have these conditions (Stimpson & Peek, 2005). A history of hypertension, arthritis and cancer in the husband was associated with increased odds for the wife to have these conditions (Stimpson & Peek, 2005). It is thought that the reciprocal influence that the partners have on each other may be due to shared living arrangements, diets, lifestyles and other shared health risks (Stimpson & Peek, 2005).

While marital type relationships are known to enhance physical health, issues related to masculinity and social connectedness can impact the mental health of men (McKenzie, Collings, Jenkin & River, 2018). McKenzie et al. (2018) suggest that when thinking about men's mental health, researchers and providers need to think about the social practices and gender relations that lead to poor mental health outcomes instead of focusing only on men with a mental health diagnosis. Men's mental health outcomes are less likely to be informed by being male, but by the social contexts men find themselves in and the types of relationships they have. Social expectations can cause men to not seek social support from other men, holding in their feelings and problems. Or men who do reach out may be shunned by others who feel that sharing personal issues and feelings shows a lack of masculinity (McKenzie et al., 2018). The general related social norming of what is and is not appropriate for a man can have significant impact on men's mental health by creating barriers to having close friendships with other men.

Men's social connectedness was shown to be a predictor of longevity in a comparative study of men in Japan and England using data from the Japan Gerontological Evaluation Study (JAGES) and the English Longitudinal Study of Ageing (ELSA) (Aida et al., 2018). The impact of family-based social relations was stronger among ELSA men, the prevalence of being married was higher among JAGES men, therefore the higher prevalence of being married seemed to add 105.4 days longevity to those in JAGES compared to ELSA (Aida et al., 2018). For ELSA men, not being underweight, non-daily drinking, not smoking and better friendship-based social relationships contributed to higher survival compared to JAGES men (Aida et al., 2018). Therefore, a lack of friends contributed to 45.4 fewer days of survival in JAGES as compared to ELSA (Aida et al., 2018).

Being in a relationship has the benefit of peer positive social controls (Houle et al., 2017) which are significantly associated with six health behaviors including health responsibility, nutrition, physical activity, interpersonal relations, stress management and spirituality. This is done through three mechanisms – shared activities such as physical activity or shared meals, being inspired by others practicing positive health behaviors and serving as a positive role model for others (Houle et al., 2017). Friends and co-workers play a significant role in promoting health behaviors among men and can be role models and influencers for adopting behaviors that support good health.

Another study on men's relationships shows that among persons with low quantity, and sometimes low quality relationships, there is an increased risk of death due to social isolation and this is a risk factor for mortality from a wide array of causes (House, Landis & Umberson, 1988). Relationship breakdowns are linked to suicide ideation and completion for men (Scourfield & Evans, 2015). This could be due to a number of factors including the changing nature of intimacy, loss of honor, marriage being a more positive experience for men than women, loss of control in the relationship and lack of men's social networks. Marital status has also shown to be an important factor for men's mortality later in life, to the point that being widowed or divorced for more than two years raises the mortality risk for men and that uncaring and unhelpful spousal behaviors outweighed the positive spousal influences, resulting in poorer overall health (Bulanda, Brown & Yamashita, 2016; Robards, Evandrou, Falkingham & Vlachantoni, 2012).

A 2017 Danish study found similar long-term health impacts of being in a same-sex marriage to the current research findings (Tatangelo, McCabe, Campbell & Szoeke, 2017). In the three decades since same-sex marriage was legalized in 1989, those in same-sex marriages showed elevated mortality during the first decade. Since 2000, however, mortality among same-sex married men has dropped to a level below that of unmarried and divorced men (Tatangelo et al., 2017). This suggests that over time there have been changes in the nature and quality of same-sex relationships, with potential impacts from changing social acceptance. A study of both straight and same-sex married couples in the United States showed that spouses in same-sex marriages played a role in influencing positive health behaviors in their partners, similar to what was found in straight marriages (Umberson, Donnelly & Pollitt, 2018).

Conclusions

Humans were created to be in relationships with each other and, as the data has consistently shown, men need to be in relationship with others for their own health. Men who place a high priority on independence and solitude consistently have worse health outcomes than men who are involved in interpersonal relationships such as marriage, close friendships and being involved with their community. Mutual trust, communication and conflict resolution are the foundation for relationships of all types, whether within a family, a workplace or in a community organization.

Future research in relationships is needed to fully understand the reasons that couples stay together despite all the challenges that can tear couples apart. Likewise, additional education for young men needs to focus on developing compassion and empathy for others, such as the challenges that girls go through during adolescence and young adulthood and how the actions of men can impact them both in the short and long term as it relates to abuse, self-esteem and self-efficacy.

Expanding beyond the individual relationships of family and friends, being in a relationship with others through community institutions and organizations creates a solid foundation of social support that is crucial to the long-term health of the individuals, institutions and the communities themselves. Working together for mutual goals that benefit the community as a whole can benefit the individual as well, which requires that we become reconnected with friends and neighbors instead of being strangers living on the same street.

In his own words

While many have heard of James Brown, either the singer or the athlete, not many have heard of James Wallis Brown (1928–2005) a petroleum engineer turned educator in the small rural Texas town of Ogelsby. Mr. Brown was born and raised in Wortham, Texas, before moving and finishing high school eight miles down the road in Mexia, Texas. He was raised in a family of six (five brothers and a sister), and while he was a lifelong bachelor, he stayed close to his immediate and extended family members, built lifelong friendships and was active in the life of his community. While Mr. Brown's life would seem to be textbook for premature mortality, he lived longer than his brothers – dying at the age of 76 – who were also lifelong bachelors (though one did marry later in life and died a few years afterwards) and second to his younger sister who was the only sibling to marry and have a family. His life was full of relationships – spending time with his brothers and cousins at the family home in Mexia; spending time with his sister, brother-in-law, nephews and grand-niece and nephew at their homes; developing relationships with students and families in Ogelsby where he worked for 27 years as a teacher, principal and superintendent before retiring two years before his death. He was known for "adopting" students with coats and school supplies magically showing up in classrooms for students whose families were struggling financially, as well as helping a few students become the first in their family to attend college. While he was not married, he created those close relationships with those he cared for and was surrounded by people who cared for him, thus having some of the same protective benefits that come from being married or in a similar relationship. As compared to his brothers, his life was longer and relatively free of health problems, outside of watching his diet due to a family history of heart disease. Mr. Brown's life, like all men's, was for a finite number of years but his legacy, due to his relationships, will last generations.

References

Aida, J., Cable, N., Zaninotto, P., Tsuboya, T., Tsakos, G., Matsuyama, Y., … & Watt, R. G. (2018). Social and behavioural determinants of the difference in survival among older adults in Japan and England. *Gerontology, 64*(3), 266–277.

Ashida, S., & Heaney, C. A. (2008). Differential associations of social support and social connectedness with structural features of social networks and the health status of older adults. *Journal of Aging and Health, 20*(7), 872–893.

Bowen, C. E., & Luy, M. (2016). Community social characteristics and health at older ages: Evidence from 156 religious communities. *The Journals of Gerontology: Series B, 73*(8), 1429–1438.

Bulanda, J. R., Brown, J. S., & Yamashita, T. (2016). Marital quality, marital dissolution, and mortality risk during the later life course. *Social Science & Medicine, 165*, 119–127.

Cohen, S., Brissette, I., Skoner, D. P., & Doyle, W. J. (2000). Social integration and health: The case of the common cold. *Journal of Social Structure, 1*(3), 1–7.

Common English Bible. (2011). *Common English Bible.* Nashville, TN: Common English Bible.

Ebrahim, S., Wannamethee, G., McCallum, A., Walker, M., & Shaper, A. G. (1995). Marital status, change in marital status, and mortality in middle-aged British men. *American Journal of Epidemiology, 142*(8), 834–842.

Goldman, N., Korenman, S., & Weinstein, R. (1995). Marital status and health among the elderly. *Social Science & Medicine, 40*(12), 1717–1730.

Gottman, J., & Levenson R. (1999). What predicts change in marital interaction over time? A study of alternative models. *Family Process, 38*(2), 143–158.

Gottman, J., & Levenson, R. (2002). A two-factor model for predicting when a couple will divorce: Exploratory analyses using a 14-year longitudinal data. *Family Process, 41*(1), 83–96.

Gottman, J. M., Levenson, R. W., Swanson, C., Swanson, K., Tyson, R., & Yoshimoto, D. (2003). Observing gay, lesbian and heterosexual couples' relationships: Mathematical modeling of conflict interaction. *Journal of Homosexuality, 45*(1), 65–91.

The Gottman Institute. (2019). *The Gottman Institute: A research-based approach to relationships.* Retrieved from www.gottman.com/

Greif, G. (2008). *Buddy System: Understanding male friendships.* Oxford: Oxford University Press.

Health Promotion Staff, Hall Health Center Health Promotion. (2014). *Healthy vs unhealthy relationships. University of Washington Hall Health Center.* http://depts.washington.edu/hhpccweb/health-resource/healthy-vs-unhealthy-relationships/

Horwitz, A. V., White, H. R., & Howell-White, S. (1996). Becoming married and mental health: A longitudinal study of a cohort of young adults. *Journal of Marriage and the Family, 58*(4), 895–907.

Houle, J., Meunier, S., Coulombe, S., Mercerat, C., Gaboury, I., Tremblay, G., … & Lavoie, B. (2017). Peer positive social control and men's health-promoting behaviors. *American Journal of Men's Health, 11*(5), 1569–1579.

House, J. S., Landis, K. R., & Umberson, D. (1988). Social relationships and health. *Science, 241*(4865), 540–545.

Jacques-Tiura, A. J., Abbey, A., Wegner, R., Pierce, J., Pegram, S. E., & Woerner, J. (2015). Friends matter: Protective and harmful aspects of male friendships associated with past-year sexual aggression in a community sample of young men. *American Journal of Public Health, 105*(5), 1001–1007.

Kaplan, R. M., & Kronick, R. G. (2006). Marital status and longevity in the United States population. *Journal of Epidemiology & Community Health, 60*(9), 760–765.

McKenzie, S. K., Collings, S., Jenkin, G., & River, J. (2018). Masculinity, social connectedness, and mental health: Men's diverse patterns of practice. *American Journal of Men's Health, 12*(5), 1247–1261.

Ramezankhani, A., Azizi, F., & Hadaegh, F. (2019). Associations of marital status with diabetes, hypertension, cardiovascular disease and all-cause mortality: A long term follow-up study. *PloS one, 14*(4), e0215593.

Robards, J., Evandrou, M., Falkingham, J., & Vlachantoni, A. (2012). Marital status, health and mortality. *Maturitas, 73*(4), 295–299.

Schoenborn, C. (2004). *Marital Status and Health: United States, 1999–2002.* Atlanta, GA: Center for Disease Control and Prevention, National Center for Health Statistics.

Scourfield, J., & Evans, R. (2015). Why might men be more at risk of suicide after a relationship breakdown? Sociological insights. *American Journal of Men's Health, 9*(5), 380–384.

Schultz, W. M., Hayek, S. S., Samman Tahhan, A., Ko, Y. A., Sandesara, P., Awad, M., … & Topel, M. L. (2017). Marital status and outcomes in patients with cardiovascular disease. *Journal of the American Heart Association, 6*(12), e005890.

Stimpson, J. P., & Peek, M. K. (2005). Concordance of chronic conditions in older Mexican American couples. *Preventing Chronic Disease, 2*(3).

Tatangelo, G., McCabe, M., Campbell, S., & Szoeke, C. (2017). Gender, marital status and longevity. *Maturitas, 100*, 64–69.

Umberson, D., Donnelly, R., & Pollitt, A. M. (2018). Marriage, social control, and health behavior: A dyadic analysis of same-sex and different-sex couples. *Journal of Health and Social Behavior, 59*(3), 429–446.

10 Fatherhood

Stephen Howes

Definition

There are many types of relationships that exist between men and their children across the globe. Despite the lack of a universal definition of the term father, the majority of men will be identified as a father at some point in their life (MenCare, 2019). According to the Child Welfare Information Gateway (2018, p. 2), the term *legal father* "generally refers to a man married to the mother at the time of conception or birth of the child or whose paternity has been otherwise determined by a court of competent jurisdiction."

While that has been the traditional legal definition, "(n)ot all men are biological fathers and not all fathers have biological children" (Jones & Mosher, 2013, p. 3). For example, a man may raise children from their partner's previous relationship if they are living together and not married, referred to as cohabitation. Some men become fathers through the legal process of adoption, by marrying their partner who has children from a previous relationship (Jones & Mosher, 2013), or with assistance from a gestational carrier. According to the U.S. Census Bureau (2018), more than half of men in the United States are fathers to biological, step, or adopted children (Figure 10.1).

A man is presumed to be the father of a child under specific circumstances in more than half of the states in the United States, such as by being listed on the child's birth certificate, by confirming he is the father of the child in writing, or by marrying "the child's mother and the child is born during the marriage or within 300 days after the marriage ended" (Child Welfare Information Gateway, 2018, p. 2). In 2015, the U.S. Supreme Court upheld the right for same-sex couples to marry. In 2017, the case of *Pavan v. Smith* clarified that the 2015 ruling extended to parenting rights. This means that children born to same-sex couples are to have the names of both parents listed on the birth certificate. Despite this ruling, LGBTQ families continue to face discrimination across the United States (American Bar Association, 2019).

Did you know?

Founded in 1994, the National Fatherhood Initiative is one of the nation's leading non-profit organizations addressing the lack of father involvement in children's lives and providing resources for community organizations to engage fathers, such as the Friendly Father Checkup (National Fatherhood Initiative, 2016a), and resources for new and current fathers, such as educational brochures and the 24/7 Dad app, designed to keep dads organized (National Fatherhood Initiative, 2016b). Learn more at www.fatherhood.org.

Fatherly Figures: A Snapshot of Dads Today

Roughly 6 in 10 men are fathers

Of the 121 million men age 15 and over in the United States, about 75 million are fathers to biological, step or adopted children.

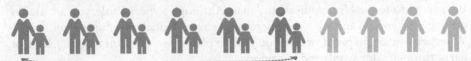

54%
of fathers have only adult children who are at least 18 years old

46%
of fathers have at least one minor child who is less than 18 years old

Roughly 1 in 4 men are grandfathers

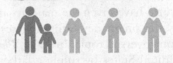

Of the 35 million fathers of minor children, 1.7 million (roughly 2 percent) are "single" fathers who are living with at least one child under 18 with no spouse or partner present.

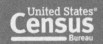

United States® Census Bureau | U.S. Department of Commerce
Economics and Statistics Administration
U.S. CENSUS BUREAU
census.gov

Source: Survey of Income and Program Participation, 2014 Panel, Wave 1
<www.census.gov/sipp/>

Figure 10.1 Fatherly figures: a snapshot of dads today.

Source: U.S. Census. Image retrieved from www.census.gov/library/visualizations/2018/comm/fathers–day.html.

Paternity

Each country and state establishes its own laws and criteria for establishing paternity. In recent decades the percentage of births to unmarried parents has increased significantly, which has led to evolving discussion and debate over fatherly rights (Child Welfare Information Gateway, 2018). As more unmarried fathers challenge custody cases, such as the termination of their parental rights when birth mothers relinquish their children for adoption, constitutional protection of a father's rights in the United States was upheld as long as a substantial relationship with his child was established (Child Welfare Information

Gateway, 2018). In these cases, the father had to demonstrate participation in raising the child and an effort in building a relationship.

According to the United States Department of Justice, child support is typically a matter addressed at the state and local levels, except in specific cases (Department of Justice, 2017). Failing to pay child support for a year is considered a criminal misdemeanor, and failing to pay child support for more than two years or owing money that exceeds $10,000 is considered a felony crime (Department of Justice, 2017).

In his own words

Jimmy Vasquez, 40. Seattle, Washington, school counselor, father
Be willing to re-establish yourself as a man. Although a special role, you are always on stage. All you do and say has a micro or macro potential to influence your child. Whether you are prepared or not, you will be placed in a position to guide, heal, or harm through your words and behaviors.

Throughout the world, a father maintains minimal rights regarding decisions of abortion (BBC, 2014). In the United States a mother does not have to gain consent from or notify the father before deciding to have an abortion. Court systems across the world have given the majority right to the mother as it is her body being most affected by the pregnancy. United States Supreme Court cases have shaped the law around this controversial topic. In 1976, *Planned Parenthood v. Danforth* gained attention across the United States by ruling a father's consent being required for a mother to undergo an abortion as unconstitutional. In 1992, *Planned Parenthood v. Casey* ruled a mother being required to notify the father of an abortion as unconstitutional as it created an undue burden and substantial obstacle for the mother that could potentially put her safety at risk.

Europe maintains abortion laws similar to the United States, including situations where parental permission may be required. According to Hofverberg (2015), women 16 and older who are requesting an abortion in Iceland are required to sign a request for an abortion. Written permission from parents is required for women who are younger, except in cases of special circumstances; however, permission from the father of the fetus is never required (Hofverberg, 2015).

Absent fathers

The National Fatherhood Initiative highlights the dramatic need for a father in a child's life (2016c). The United Nations (2017) reports that about 27% of homes globally do not have two parents living at home with their children. Specifically, "(o)ne-parent households are more prevalent in Africa, Latin America and the Caribbean, and less prevalent in Asia" (United Nations, 2017). According to the U.S. Census Bureau (2016), about one in four children in the United States live without their biological father in the home. Children raised without a father are at an increased risk for multiple health concerns ranging from behavioral problems and poverty to obesity (see Figure 10.2).

It is important for children to feel loved and supported and having a father that is knowingly absent can be emotionally, physically, mentally, and financially challenging for

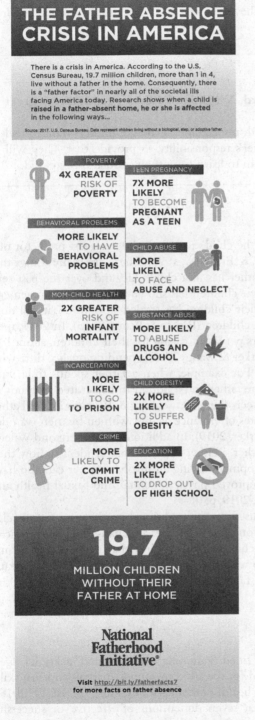

Figure 10.2 The father absence crisis in America: Infographic describing the impact of father's absence.

Source: National Fatherhood Initiative®.

children. There is a common myth that children, particularly boys, who are raised without a father are not disciplined, however research actually indicates that mothers tend to do more of the disciplining simply because they tend to spend more time with their children (Biblarz & Stacey, 2010).

In his own words

Joseph Barrett, 91. Mt. Crawford, Virginia. Father, grandfather, great grandfather
Fathers should treat their children with respect and fairness. Children want to feel loved and it is the father's and mother's responsibility to provide that. They will make mistakes as you did so teach them to learn from their mistakes, as you did.

Father involvement

The quality of the relationship between the child's parents is the strongest predictor of a father's involvement (Doherty, Kouneski, & Erickson, 1998). There are many things that can impact the level of involvement a father has in a child's life, and over the past several decades, father involvement with their children has shown promising improvement. Although the time fathers spend with their children has tripled since 1965, it still does not match the time mothers spend with children (Parker & Wang, 2013). In 2011, men were spending approximately seven hours per week caring for their children, about half the time that mothers were spending (Parker & Wang, 2013). Spending quality time with children is important for many reasons. For example, when a father spends time with their child, the child feels validated by the father and a bond can be created that aids in developing a deeper understanding between them (Rosenberg & Wilcox, 2006). Father involvement is also linked to lowering rates of violence against women by men (van der Gaag, Heilman, Gupta, Nembhard, & Barker, 2019). In addition, Rosenberg and Wilcox (2006) argue that by spending time together, a father is able to better identify how they can support the child's growth and development. Being an involved father can also have health benefits for the father, such as "improved physical, mental, and sexual health and reduced risk-taking" (van der Gaag et al., 2019, p. 9).

While much of the literature has focused on the traditional mother and father relationship, it's important to include discussion of how families are changing. The American Academy of Child and Adolescent Psychiatry (2013) shares that a child's emotional development is based on the relationship with their parents, not on their parents' sexual orientation, thereby supporting LGBT families in raising well-adjusted and healthy children.

Dimensions of fathering

In 2018, an international video campaign titled "Parenting is also learned" acknowledged the challenges of parenting and advocated for the need to support parents to learn skills for effective parenting to achieve optimal health outcomes for children (UNICEF, 2018). Rosenberg & Wilcox (2006) explain that seven dimensions of effective or successful fathering emerge from research on the topic. The seven dimensions focus on developing a relationship with the child's mother and the child, spending quality time interacting with the child, and delivering discipline calmly and consistently, while also serving as a child's role model, fostering their independence and autonomy while providing emotional security and physical safety (Rosenberg & Wilcox, 2006). While it may be difficult, and sometimes feel impossible, to master all seven dimensions, putting forth effort to all and excelling in some can have great impact on children and families (Rosenberg & Wilcox, 2006). An additional inherent key role of a father is to be a role model, which could allow him to model healthy living by making healthy food choices. It can also subconsciously model how to be an absent father.

In his own words

Gordon Stokes, 43. Alexandria, Virginia. Middle school principal and father

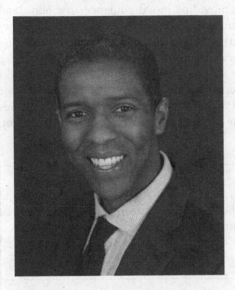

Figure 10.3 Gordon Stokes.
Source: Image provided by Karen Bolt, Fairfax County Public Schools.

My wife and I read various books on infants and early parenthood in preparation for our first child. We also took a delivery class to try and get an understanding for what to expect. Purchasing and studying our baby books prepared us for how to calm a crying child when they are five days old. Working through the constant schedule of sleep and feeding for a few months was challenging. Obviously, I could not do the heavy lifting of carrying a child. After she was born, it has been crucial to share as many responsibilities as possible. This makes parenting truly shared. Many of the skills I possess as a father come from my own father/son relationship. My dad was always present. While my mom was no-nonsense, dealing with the day-to-day foolishness, my dad was the steady presence, supporting the stability of our family. He would provide the big lessons when me or my brother needed some correction. Most importantly, he lived a great example: he worked hard throughout his life to achieve many positive things (family, career, home), he had a sense of humor, and he put the needs of the family before his own needs.

Parenting styles

Although there are many styles of parenting, researchers typically identify three primary styles: traditional, a mix of traditional and modern, and modern. This research has been typically assessed with a heteronormative approach, excluding same-sex parenting perspectives. Historically, the traditional role of a father in the household has been narrowly conceived and based on gender roles, with the primary and sole function defined by the responsibility to financially support the family (Osborne, Dillon, Winter Craver, & Hovey, 2016). Across the globe, this remains as a persistent social and cultural expectation (van der Gaag et al., 2019).

Things have been changing, and there has been a movement in some parts of the world toward a more modern parenting style. Osborne et al. (2016) further explain that a modern father is involved "in nearly every aspect of parenting from spending leisure time with his child, nurturing and caregiving, providing moral guidance, discipline, and support" (p. 6). A present and active father has been linked to increased positive outcomes in the child's cognitive development, educational achievement, and self-esteem (Osborne et al., 2016). More men across the United States are staying home from work to care for their children. Fathers who stay at home to care for their children while the mother works are commonly known as stay-at-home dads. According to Livingston (2014), the number of stay-at-home dads nearly doubled between 1989 and 2012. A parenting style that shares characteristics from both the traditional and the modern is possible as part of a parenting style continuum (see Figure 10.4).

Did you know?

National Responsible Fatherhood Clearinghouse promotes strong fathers and families by sharing research and resources about fatherhood, operating a national call center for fathers and practitioners (1-877-4DAD411), and offering free online trainings available on their website (n.d.). Learn more at www.fatherhood.gov.

Did you know?

MenCare is a global fatherhood campaign that spans 50 countries. With a mission for gender equality, MenCare works globally to promote the health of families with engaged fathers. Learn more at www.men-care.org.

Learn more

The Evolution of Dad is a documentary created by Dana H. Glazer, an American dad, about the evolution of fatherhood and the impact of this on families and society at large (2019). Learn more at www.evolutionofdad.com/.

What's your fatherhood style?

This self-assessment may help you reflect on your preferred parenting style of fatherhood. Using the scale provided, indicate your reaction to each of the following statements. After answering each statement, add up the total number of points and locate your scoring range.

1	2	3	4	5
Strongly Disagree	Disagree	Partially Agree	Agree	Strongly Agree

_____1. It is the father's role in the family to be the financial provider.

_____2. The child's mother should assume the role as the nurturing parent.

_____3. It is the father's role to teach the children lessons about hard work and earning a living.

_____4. A mother's role is to stay home with the children. A father should be working for his family.

_____5. When using discipline, a child should receive some form of punishment in order to understand wrongdoing.

_____6. When the father spends time with his children, the activity is what's most important.

_____7. Fathers who do not live at home with their children (referred to as nonresident fathers) will never have the same quality relationship with their child compared to a resident father.

_____8. When a nonresident father spends time with his children, they should engage in mostly fun and enjoyable activities.

_____9. It is not fair to ask a nonresident father to be an equal disciplinarian co-parent.

_____10. If a father does not live in the same home as his children, he should not be expected to contribute financially outside or above any legal obligation.

Scoring range results

35–50 points: This range indicates a preference for a **traditional style** of fatherhood beliefs and parental roles. This parenting philosophy supports the heteronormative belief that men are providers and women are caretakers in a family dynamic. Time fathers spend with children is usually disciplinary or work related and the father is often viewed as the less nurturing parent. Although the father takes his role very seriously, parental roles are often divided and not shared between parents.

18–34 points: This range indicates a preference for a mix of **traditional and modern style of fatherhood** beliefs and parental roles. This parenting philosophy also supports the heteronormative belief that men are providers and women are caretakers in a family dynamic. However, there is confidence in a father's ability and responsibility to nurture a child.

17 points or lower: This range indicates a preference for a **modern style of fatherhood** beliefs and parental roles. This parenting philosophy supports shared co-parenting roles and responsibilities. It is acceptable for either parent to be the primary breadwinner and supports the other parent to be a stay-at-home parent. In addition, there is confidence that a father who does not live in the same home as the child is still fully capable of fulfilling co-parenting roles and maintaining a consistent, fulfilling relationship with their child.

Figure 10.4 What's your fatherhood style?

Source: Developed by Stephen Howes from multiple sources and experiences. © 2018, Stephen Howes.

Key next steps

Advancements in what we know about being a present and involved father will only take place through increased research, education, policy, and advocacy. There are a number of significant gaps in research. For example, limited research exists on the diversity of fatherhood outside of a mother–father dynamic, such as children with two fathers. The data on fatherless children is primarily focused on children with a mother and father, and the impact of the father's absence in the child's life. For example, Biblarz and Stacey (2010) argue that the gender of parents is not as important as the quality of relationship that they have with their child and that statements indicating that, in order to thrive, children must have both a mother and father are not actually supported by research. They further argue that two adults, regardless of gender, sexual orientation or marital status, can offer more benefits to a child than one parent alone (Biblarz & Stacey, 2010). Research is also limited about single heterosexual fathers or gay fathers as a result of divorce and same-sex parents through adoption or surrogacy (Biblarz & Stacey, 2010), and also older father (Fathers.com, n.d.). Supporting, mobilizing, and utilizing national and global non-profit organizations will continue to address the needs of fathers and their children.

Currently in the United States, there are advocacy efforts for an Office on Men's Health within the federal government as an equal entity to the Office on Women's Health (Men's Health, 2015) and a White House Council on Boys and Men (Coalition to Create a White House Council on Boys and Men, n.d.). A dedicated network of the nation's leading professionals would be able to establish a commitment to current men's health issues highlighting programs and advocating for effective fathering across the country. The effective fathering of the nation's children will most successfully be accomplished one community at a time, and state and local legislation will need to find outreach programs to educate and empower men across the country. One of the places where efforts could be made to empower men is in the workplace. For example, van der Gaag et al. (2019) stress the value in workplaces of providing equal opportunities for fathers to take paid leave to care for their children.

References

American Academy of Child and Adolescent Psychiatry. (2013). *Children with lesbian, gay, bisexual and transgender parents [Fact Sheet]*. Retrieved from www.aacap.org/App_Themes/AACAP/docs/facts_for_families/92_children_with_lesbian_gay_bisexual_transgender_parents.pdf

American Bar Association. (2019). *National LGBT Bar Association Commission on Sexual Orientation and Gender Identity Report to the House of Delegates Resolution*. Retrieved from www.americanbar.org/content/dam/aba/images/news/2019mymhodres/113.pdf

BBC. (2014). *Ethics guide*. Retrieved from www.bbc.co.uk/ethics/abortion/legal/fathers.shtml

Biblarz, T. J., & Stacey, J. (2010). How does the gender of parents matter? *Journal of Marriage and Family, 72*, 3–22. doi: 10.1111/j.1741-3737.2009.00678.x

Child Welfare Information Gateway. (2018). *The rights of unmarried fathers*. Washington, DC: U.S. Department of Health and Human Services, Children's Bureau. Retrieved from www.childwelfare.gov/topics/systemwide/laws-policies/statutes/putative/

Coalition to Create a White House Council on Boys and Men. (n.d.). *About*. Retrieved from http://whitehouseboysmen.org/about

Doherty, W. J., Kouneski, E. F., & Erickson, M. F. (1998). Responsible fathering: An overview and conceptual framework. *Journal of Marriage and the Family, 60*, 277–292

The Evolution of Dad. (2019). *About*. Retrieved from www.evolutionofdad.com/about

Fathers.com. (n.d.). *Our history.* Retrieved from http://fathers.com/about-ncf/our-history/

Hofverberg, E. (2015). *Abortion legislation in Europe: Iceland.* Retrieved fromwww.loc.gov/law/help/abortion-legislation/europe.php#_ftnref55

Jones, J., & Mosher, W. (2013). Fathers' involvement with their children: United States, 2006–2010. *National Health Statistics Reports,* (71). Retrieved from www.cdc.gov/nchs/data/nhsr/nhsr071.pdf

Livingston, G. (2014). *Growing number of dads home with the kids.* Retrieved from www.pewsocialtrends.org/2014/06/05/growing-number-of-dads-home-with-the-kids/

MenCare. (2019). *About MenCare.* Retrieved from https://men-care.org/about-mencare/

Men's Health. (2015). *The most important thing you can do for your health today.* Retrieved from www.menshealth.com/health/a19548128/office-of-mens-health/

National Fatherhood Initiative. (2016a). *Father-friendly check-up.* Retrieved from www.fatherhood.org/ffcu?hsCtaTracking=896046b0-1edd-4ca8-a37a-4c572af7f864%7C3005656d-2e7c-4ccc-bb38-ffe1d0bbfedd

National Fatherhood Initiative. (2016b). *History.* Retrieved from www.fatherhood.org/history

National Fatherhood Initiative. (2016c). *The proof is in: Father absence harms children.* Retrieved from www.fatherhood.org/father-absence-statistic

National Responsible Fatherhood Clearinghouse. (n.d.). *About us.* Retrieved from www.fatherhood.gov/about-us

Osborne, C., Dillon, D., Winter Craver, J., & Hovey, I. (2016). *Making good on fatherhood: A review of the fatherhood research.* Child and Family Research Partnership. Retrieved from https://cdn2.hubspot.net/hubfs/135704/CFRPReport_MakingGoodonFathers_ReviewofPgmResearch.pdf

Parker, K., & Wang, W. (2013). *Modern parenthood: Roles of moms and dads converge as they balance work and family.* Pew Research Center, *Social & Demographic Trends.* Retrieved from www.pewsocialtrends.org/2013/03/14/modern-parenthood-roles-of-moms-and-dads-converge-as-they-balance-work-and-family/

Pavan v. Smith, 137 S. Ct. 2075 (2017)

Planned Parenthood v. Danforth, 428 U.S. 52 (1976)

Planned Parenthood v. Casey, 505 U.S. 833 (1992)

Rosenberg, J., & Wilcox, W. B. (2006). *The importance of fathers in the healthy development of children.* Retrieved from www.childwelfare.gov/pubpdfs/fatherhood.pdf

UNICEF. (2018). *"Parenting is also learned" campaign launched to help parents raise happy, healthy and smart children.* Retrieved from www.unicef.org/northmacedonia/press-releases/parenting-also-learned-campaign-launched-help-parents-raise-happy-healthy-and-smart

United Nations. (2017). *Household size and composition around the world 2017.* Retrieved from www.un.org/en/development/desa/population/publications/pdf/ageing/household_size_and_composition_around_the_world_2017_data_booklet.pdf

U.S. Census Bureau. (2016). *C3. Living arrangements of children under 18 years and marital status of parents, by age, sex, race, and Hispanic origin and selected characteristics of the child for all children: 2016.* Retrieved from www.census.gov/data/tables/2016/demo/families/cps-2016.html

U.S. Census Bureau. (2018). *Fatherly figures: A snapshot of dads today.* Retrieved from www.census.gov/library/visualizations/2018/comm/fathers-day.html

U.S. Department of Justice. (2017). *Citizen's guide to U.S. federal law on child support enforcement.* Retrieved from www.justice.gov/criminal-ceos/citizens-guide-us-federal-law-child-support-enforcement

van der Gaag, N., Heilman, B., Gupta, T., Nembhard, C., & Barker, G. (2019). *State of the World's Fathers: Unlocking the power of men's care.* Washington, DC: Promundo-US. Retrieved from https://stateoftheworldsfathers.org/report/state-of-the-worlds-fathers-helping-men-step-up-to-care/

11 Violence

Sara K. Fehr and Diana Karczmarczyk

There are many types of violence that people can commit against others. This chapter will focus primarily on domestic violence, sometimes referred to as intimate partner violence, sexual harassment, and sexual abuse. These are all of critical importance to be included in a book on men's health because men are both perpetrators and victims of these types of violence.

Intimate partner violence

Intimate partner violence is a global public health crisis. It pervades all segments of society regardless of an individual's race, ethnicity, age, sexual orientation, country of origin, or sex. While violence against men poses a serious threat to health and wellbeing, women are disproportionately impacted by sexual violence, stalking, and intimate partner violence (Breiding et al., 2014). Intimate partner violence perpetrated against women by men is one of the most common types of violence around the globe (Garcia-Moreno, Guedes, & Knerr, 2012).

Violence against women often occurs when women do not live and practice within the bounds of expected gender roles/norms (Heise, Ellsberg, & Gottmoeller, 2002). These roles and norms may include women staying in the home, women raising children, women acting subservient to men, modest standards of dress, and interaction with males outside the family. This global issue is found in countries such as Bangladesh, India, Mexico, Nigeria, Zimbabwe, and many more (Heise, Ellsberg, & Gottmoeller, 1999). Because these cultural norms exist, it is challenging to raise awareness about these types of abuse as well as garner community support for efforts to end violence against women.

Although violence against women is well studied, little information exists on the worldwide burden of violence against men. This is likely due to the fact that (1) men are less likely to report instances of intimate partner violence and (2) traditional cultural practices that often justify violence against women may not see violence against men as an issue.

Consider this

Why do you think that men are less likely to report instances of intimate partner violence?

There are four main types of behaviors that can be characterized as part of intimate partner violence. These include physical violence, sexual violence, stalking, and psychological aggression (Centers for Disease Control and Prevention [CDC], 2019). In the United States alone, it is estimated that nearly 10% of men, 15 million, have been sexually assaulted, physically assaulted, or stalked by an intimate partner (CDC, 2019). The CDC (2019) reports that 38 million men, compared to 43 million women, experienced psychological aggression in their lifetime by an intimate partner who used verbal and/or non-verbal communication to cause emotional harm or to exert control over them.

The 2019 Crime Survey for England and Wales indicates that 4.2% of men (786,000) experienced domestic violence in the prior year (Office for National Statistics, 2019). However, in Canada, 2014 data indicated that men and women equally reported domestic violence, referred to as spousal violence, although men were slightly less likely to report to the police than women (The Canadian Centre for Justice Statistics, 2016). This difference in data may be indicative of changes in reporting behaviors.

According to the CDC (2019), consequences of domestic violence include "conditions affecting the heart, digestive, reproductive, muscle and bones, and nervous systems, many of which are chronic in nature" (para. 8). These conditions don't just happen as the violence is occurring, but can impact a person throughout their lives (World Health Organization, United Nations Development Programme, & United Nations Office on Drugs and Crime, 2014). Male victims, like female victims, may feel unsafe or fearful, experience symptoms of post-traumatic stress disorder, endure physical injuries, and need assistance for various social services (Breiding et al., 2014).

Did you know?

The ManKind Initiative (2014) created an advertisement that has received more than 8 million views promoting the message that domestic violence perpetrated by women on men is also violence, indicated by the #violenceisviolence tag. Watch the advertisement at www.youtube.com/watch?v=u3PgH86OyEM.

Did you know?

There are several national domestic violence hotlines, with corresponding websites, in the United States (National Resource Center on Domestic Violence, n.d.). These include:

1. National Domestic Violence Hotline
   Website: www.thehotline.org
   Phone: 800-799-SAFE (7233)

2. StrongHearts Native Helpline (dedicated to serving Native Americans)
   Website: www.strongheartshelpline.org/
   Phone: 1-844-762-8483

Many other countries offer their own hotline to provide support for those experiencing domestic violence and their information is also available online.

Sexual harassment

Sexual harassment in the workplace has been recognized globally as a significant health issue causing leaders in the United Nations (2017) to address the pervasive and detrimental nature of this type of violence. Furthermore, in 2018, Actionaid.org reported that 50% of women who experienced sexual harassment believed it "would be pointless" to report it to the police because of its pervasiveness, and cited concerns about effective responses (para. 1). Sexual harassment includes unwelcome sexual advances, requests for sexual favors, and other verbal or physical harassment of a sexual nature. Though it can happen to anyone, sexual harassment experienced by men is not as widely reported or studied as compared to sexual harassment experienced by women (Bailey, 2018). The U.S. Equal Employment Opportunity Commission (n.d.) reports sexual harassment claims filed with their agency and these indicate that between 2010 and 2018 the rate of claims by men has ranged between 15.9 and 16.7%, with the highest percentage in 2013. This indicates a consistent challenge in the workplace for men.

As with other data on violence, sexual harassment experienced by men in the workplace may also be underreported. One limitation to reporting may be that men may have different perceptions of how they perceive or define sexual harassment (Bailey, 2018). When sexual harassment is studied, the data indicates that men also experience harassment in the workplace, at rates that may seem surprising. In a research study of 522 workers, McLaughlin, Uggen, and Blackstone (2012) reported that 58% of females and 37% of males in a supervisory role reported experiencing harassment in a male-dominated workplace. Furthermore, they found that males in a non-supervisory role experienced slightly more harassment than females in a non-supervisory role. For men in a non-supervisory role in a male-dominated workplace, 36% experienced harassment compared to 32% of females (McLaughlin et al., 2012). In a female-dominated workplace, 35% of men experienced harassment compared to 32% of females (McLaughlin et al., 2012).

In a survey of 326 men, men were more likely to experience sexual harassment in a workplace if the men engaged in feminist activism and tolerated sexual harassment (Holland, Rabelo, Gustafson, Seabrook, & Cortina, 2016). Therefore, Holland et al. argued that men who did not align with traditional masculinity were essentially subjected to sexual harassment in the workplace as punishment, prompting recommendations for comprehensive training to prevent sexual harassment of all employees in the workplace.

Sexual abuse

In the 2006 World Report on Violence against Children, global estimates were that 73 million boys and 150 million girls experienced sexual violence with physical contact to include forced sexual intercourse and child sexual abuse (Pinheiro, 2006). Research has found that men who are sexually assaulted are often young, single, and report having physical, emotional, and/or intellectual disabilities (Stermac, del Bove, & Addison, 2004). A study of more than 34,000 adults in the United States indicated that childhood sexual abuse (CSA) had been experienced by one in ten people in their lifetime (Pérez-Fuentes et al., 2013). Specifically, CSA was experienced by 24.8% of men and by 75.2% of women, indicating a prevalence three times higher in women than men (Pérez-Fuentes et al., 2013). Despite these significant figures, most researchers still believe that the number of people who experience sexual violence, specifically CSA, is even higher due to under-reporting of sexual violence incidents. Under-reporting may be due in part to the fact that masculinity is often associated with power and control, so being a victim of sexual violence as a male may carry a deep sense of emasculation (Kapur & Muddell, 2016) and this comes with additional shame and stigma.

Learn more

Boys and Men Healing is a documentary film featuring three men who share their stories of childhood sexual abuse (BigVoice Pictures, 2019). To learn about the film or about resources available to support those who have experienced sexual abuse, visit http://bigvoicepictures.com/production-3/boys-and-men-healing/.

Violence among and by men

An important question to consider is why men and boys continue to perpetuate violence toward others. Some experts believe that the "man box" promotes messages of violence among and by men. Inspired by the work of Paul Kivel, Glickman (2012) explains that masculinity is performative and describes acting in the "man box." In the United States, a man is usually described as strong, a heterosexual, and someone who drinks alcohol and shows limited emotions (Glickman, 2012). The descriptors that are offered are uniform and common because there is an expectation that men in the United States appear and behave according to a strict code that places them in a box, with limited flexibility or diversity of expectations. Glickman argues that "the performance of masculinity requires constant vigilance to make sure that nobody sees any missteps. Since the logic of the box is an either/or, you're either all the way in or you're all the way out" (2012, para. 3). Men that do not perform according to the expectations cast as part of the man box are often labeled as "gay," "weak" or a "loser" (Glickman, 2012, para. 2). Furthermore, Glickman describes the box as follows:

> Since the Box is hierarchical as well as performative, the guy at the bottom of the heap is at risk of being cast out. So each guy has to compete with the others in order to not be the one who's outside the Box. And as each one's performance becomes more vigorous, it forces the others to do the same.
>
> (2012, para. 5)

It is this concept of competition, internally and externally, to behave and be accepted that drives behaviors that are not supportive of men expressing vulnerabilities, emotions, and their true selves with each other.

In his own words

James Landrith, 49. Alexandria, Virginia. Survivor of sexual assault, civil liberties and victim advocate

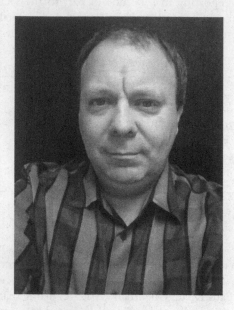

Figure 11.1 James Landrith.
Source: Image provided by James Landrith.

Men are taught at a young age to idealize figures like Chuck Norris. So, if a man is a victim of any type of violence, it is their fault. It is always your fault. You need to be more violent than your offender, if you are not – then you are weak. There is never any guilt or pushback on the offender. I was often the smallest and youngest kid in class and I was bullied both verbally and physically. It was never my bully's fault. It was always mine. If only I had fought back harder, then it would never have happened to me. So, it's ironic when people ask why men don't talk about this because the message has always been clear – it's our fault … always. No one calls out the bully or their parents if they condone this type of behavior at home. The onus is always on the victim, not the bully. There is no support for men to be their authentic selves. We just put a band-aid on these situations. This creates trauma that lasts a lifetime. This is why I fight for people who are ignored.

Learn more

Written by the internationally recognized TED Talk speaker, Tony Porter, *Breaking Out of the "Man Box"* explores how men are socialized on what it means to be a man (Skyhorse Publishing, 2019). To learn about the book, visit www.skyhorsepublishing. com/9781510701496/breaking-out-of-the-man-box/.

Hate crimes

Hate crimes are increasingly becoming an issue in the United States as biases and fear against those who do not fit the white heteronormative standard grows. These unfounded biases may then become grounds for violence against others in the form of a hate crime. According to federal law, a hate crime is one "motivated by bias against race, color, religion, national origin, sexual orientation, gender, gender identity, or disability" (U.S. Department of Justice [USDOJ], n.d., para. 8). While the sex of offenders is often not included in hate crime statistics, we do know that from 2016 to 2017, the number of hate crimes reported increased by 17% with 5,060 crimes committed on the basis of race, ethnicity or ancestry (American Bar Association [ABA], 2019; U.S. Department of Justice–Federal Bureau of Investigation [USDOJFBI], n.d.). Racial and ethnic biases motivated nearly 49% of anti-Black and 11% of anti-Hispanic hate crimes. Among the 1,338 victims of hate crimes due to bias against sexual orientation, 58% were targeted due to offenders' anti-gay bias (USDOJFBI, n.d.). This equates to roughly 2,480 blacks and 555 Hispanic individuals being targeted, and 775 men being attacked because they were gay. These reported numbers are exceedingly low as there are an estimated 250,000 hate crimes committed a year in the United States (USDOJ, n.d.). Individuals might not come forward to report they have been victims of hate crimes due to their immigration status, fear of deportation (ABA, 2019), fear, and shame.

Current efforts

Bystander intervention programs exist to combat violence on college campuses in the United States. For example, the Men's Project reinforces men's roles in sexual assault prevention by tackling issues such as "gender socialization, male privilege, and sexuality, followed by a few weeks exploring the breadth and depth of sexual violence, including its emotional and psychological impacts on survivors" (Stewart, 2014, p. 481). This program has been shown to increase men's willingness to act as a bystander, confidence in being a bystander, and acting as remits advocates (Stewart, 2014). Other programs, such as Green Dot, strive to end domestic violence, stalking, and sexual assault on college campuses (Alteristic.org, n.d.). This approach teaches both men and women the skills to intervene when they believe power-based personal violence is imminent. This approach has been shown to reduce rates of intimate partner violence on participating college campuses (Alteristic.org, n.d.). If a student has already been the victim of violence, many college campuses offer a multitude of resources through student assistance services, health services, university police, and counseling services offices. These services are designed to support both the mental and physical health of the student.

There have been several educational campaigns created to raise awareness of violence against men. One of these, called *No more excuses*, consisted of print ads and videos that were created by Joyful Heart, Viacom and 1in6 in 2016 (Joyful Heart Foundation, 2019). The campaign was designed to provide both information and support for those adult men who were sexually abused as children (Joyful Heart Foundation, 2019). See Figure 11.2 for an example of one of the print ads.

Key next steps

Global efforts to reduce violence against women perpetrated by men are complex and require an expansive, culturally competent response. Cultural competence is key to understanding and combating violence. Pan et al. (2006) investigated the *Ahimsa for Safe Families Project*; a program addressing domestic violence in Latino, Vietnamese, and Somali immigrant communities. Table 11.1 represents their key findings for these specific cultures.

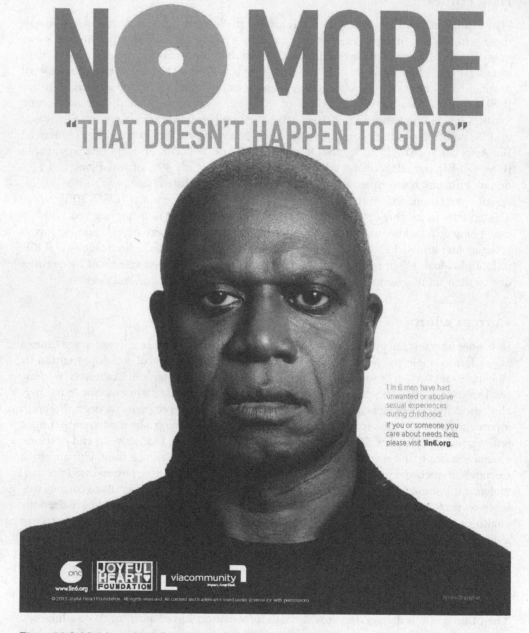

Figure 11.2 NoMore_ANDRE.jpg. Andre Braugher is featured as part of the NO MORE Excuses: The male survivors campaign series.

Source: Image developed by Joyful Heart in 2016.

These findings from the *Ahimsa for Safe Families Project* may be extrapolated to other unique and diverse populations. First, different communities have differing definitions for domestic violence, with emphasis on intergenerational and physical violence (Pan et al., 2006). This poses a global challenge as different cultures might not recognize emotional abuse, verbal abuse, sexual abuse, and stalking as domestic violence. Cultural norms exist

Table 11.1 Cultural views of domestic violence against women for Latino, Vietnamese, and Somali immigrant communities

Community	Cultural views of domestic violence against women
Latino	• Physical/verbal abuse not acceptable • Common stressors for domestic violence include economics, immigration status, and substance use
Vietnamese	• Private family problem • Physical violence not acceptable • Seeking outside help for domestic violence not acceptable • Most common stressor for domestic violence is economics
Somali	• Domestic violence only includes physical violence • Physical violence is not acceptable to resolve conflict • Physical violence is acceptable to maintain traditional family gender norms • Common stressors for domestic violence include changing gender roles post-immigration and cultural norms

Source: Adapted from Pan et al. (2006).

which might support traditional gender roles where men control and discipline their families through threats and force. Second, barriers to combating domestic violence include the lack of bilingual and bicultural resources (Pan et al., 2006). Within the boundaries of a given region there may be multiple languages spoken and multiple cultures present. If these languages and cultures are not represented in both preventative and reactionary resources, individuals might not be able to relate to or access these programs.

In 2016, member states at the World Health Assembly endorsed a global plan, "strengthening the role of the health systems in addressing interpersonal violence, in particular against women and girls and against children" (World Health Organization, 2017, para. 22). For high-income countries, they suggested advocacy, counseling, improving access, and healthcare outreach as strategies to both prevent and address intimate partner violence. In low-income areas with fewer resources, they suggested preventing violence through female economic and social empowerment, promoting healthy relationships, reducing alcohol use, and challenging traditional gender norms which place women on a lower social status than men (World Health Organization, 2017).

Resources and services must be provided at the college, state, national, and global levels to ensure access to resources and programs. In the United States, at the state and national levels, the Domestic Violence Resource Network (DVRN) is funded by the Family Violence Prevention and Service Act to strengthen domestic violence prevention and intervention through multiple national, special issue, culturally specific, and emerging issue resource centers (National Resource Center on Domestic Violence [NRCDV], n.d.). At the collegiate level, the U.S. Department of Education's Office of Civil Rights (2015) enforces legislation to address all forms of violence on college campuses. Title IX of the Education Amendment states, "no person in the United States shall, on the basis of sex, be excluded from participation in, be denied the benefits of, or be subjected to discrimination under any education program or activity receiving Federal financial assistance." (U.S. Department of Education, 2015, para. 2) In short, this amendment prohibits sexual assault, sexual harassment, and discrimination on the basis of sex. Schools must have policies and procedures in place to investigate any allegations of these forms of violence and sanction students who have been found responsible for violating Title IX (U.S. Department of Education, 2015).

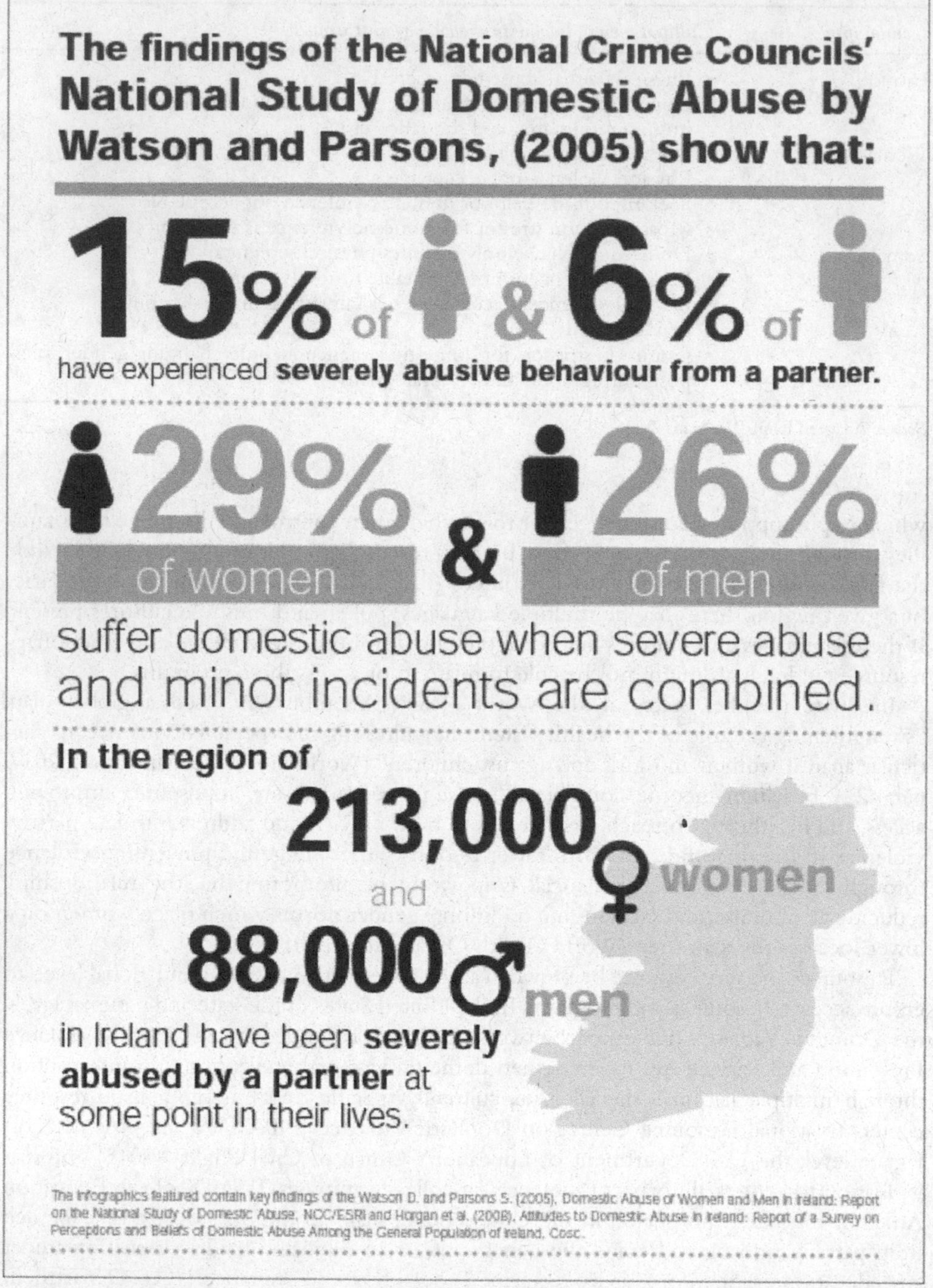

The findings of the National Crime Councils'
National Study of Domestic Abuse by
Watson and Parsons, (2005) show that:

15% of 👤 & 6% of 👤

have experienced **severely abusive behaviour from a partner.**

👤 **29%** & 👤 **26%**

of women & of men

suffer domestic abuse when severe abuse
and minor incidents are combined.

In the region of

213,000 ♀ women
and
88,000 ♂ men

in Ireland have been **severely**
abused by a partner at
some point in their lives.

The infographics featured contain key findings of the Watson D. and Parsons S. (2005), Domestic Abuse of Women and Men in Ireland: Report on the National Study of Domestic Abuse, NCC/ESRI and Horgan et al. (2008), Attitudes to Domestic Abuse in Ireland: Report of a Survey on Perceptions and Beliefs of Domestic Abuse Among the General Population of Ireland, Cosc.

Figure 11.3 Findings of the National Crime Councils' National Study of Domestic Abuse. This infographic depicts the outcomes of multiple data sources identified in the figure.

Source: Image developed by Cosc. Cosc is the National Office for the Prevention of Domestic, Sexual and Gender-based Violence.

In May 2019, Ireland announced the launch of a new hotline available for men and boys who may be experiencing domestic violence (Aodha, 2019). The initial goal for the hotline is to support 5,000 callers since reports indicate that as many as 88,000 men in Ireland report experiencing domestic violence in their lives (Aodha, 2019) (see Figure 11.3).

However, global efforts to support men experiencing domestic violence face significant challenges, such as insufficient funding and staffing. For example, the ManKind Initiative (2019) in the UK began in 2001 to provide support and services to male survivors with a small part time labor force and several volunteers. Over the years they have sought help from the public to continue their services (ManKind Initiative, 2019). For the past few years, the organization has seen a decline in financial support likely due to most funds being diverted to programs that only support women, not men, as survivors of violence (Wells, 2015).

Furthermore, there is concern by some leading global organizations that engaging men in the work to reduce violence against women is not addressing the global patriarchy and gender inequalities that exist, rather it centers men, further perpetuating male dominance (Apolitical.co, 2018). Kapur and Muddell (2016) suggest that there is a "tendency to conflate sexual violence with violence against women and girls, which contributes to the perception that it is a women's issue, thus limiting the responses available to victims falling outside of this group, including men and boys" (p. 1).

As part of ongoing joint collaborations, UN Women and MenEngage released a joint report that outlines strategies to address gender equity (MenCare & UN Women, 2014). Recommendations from MenCare & UN Women (2014) include engaging men to "be actively committed to redistributing power in both their personal lives and in larger spheres" (p. 3) and "implement policies, as well [as] campaigns to transform perceptions of gender roles among men" (p. 4). UN Women also launched the global campaign, HeForShe, to raise awareness for and end gender inequality by including men and boys in the movement (UN Women, 2014).

Did you know?

You can join HeForShe and commit to ending gender-based bias, violence, and discrimination so that people of all genders are treated equally (HeForShe.org, 2019). To learn more, visit www.heforshe.org.

References

Actionaid.org. (2018). Women say reporting sexual harassment is "pointless". Retrieved from www.actionaid.org.uk/latest-news/women-say-reporting-sexual-harassment-is-pointless

Alteristic.org. (n.d.). *Green Dot for college campuses.* Retrieved from https://alteristic.org/services/green-dot/green-dot-colleges/

American Bar Association. (2019). Midyear 2019: Why are hate crimes rising? Retrieved from www.americanbar.org/news/abanews/aba-news-archives/2019/01/midyear-2019--why-are-hate-crimes-rising-/

Aodha, G. N. (2019). *A new helpline for male victims of domestic abuse has been launched today.* Retrieved from www.thejournal.ie/male-victims-domestic-abuse-helpline-4643294-May2019/

Apolitical.co. (2018). *Men are at the root of violence. But should prevention focus on them?* Retrieved from https://apolitical.co/solution_article/men-root-violence-prevention-focus/

Bailey, R. (2018). *Many men are sexually harassed in the workplace – so why aren't they speaking out?* Retrieved from https://theconversation.com/many-men-are-sexually-harassed-in-the-workplace-so-why-arent-they-speaking-out-93081

Big Voice Pictures. (2019). *Boys and men healing*. Retrieved from http://bigvoicepictures.com/production-3/boys-and-men-healing/

Breiding, M. J., Smith, S. G., Basile, K. C., Walters, M. L., Chen, J., & Merrick, M. T. (2014). Prevalence and characteristics of sexual violence, stalking, and intimate partner violence victimization: national intimate partner and sexual violence survey, United States, 2011. *Morbidity and Mortality Weekly Report. Surveillance Summaries* (Washington, DC: 2002), *63*(8), 1–18.

Canadian Centre for Justice Statistics. (2016). *Family violence in Canada: A statistical profile, 2014.* Retrieved from www150.statcan.gc.ca/n1/pub/85-002-x/2016001/article/14303-eng.pdf

Centers for Disease Control and Prevention. (2019). *Preventing intimate partner violence.* Retrieved from www.cdc.gov/violenceprevention/intimatepartnerviolence/fastfact.html

Garcia-Moreno, C., Guedes, A., & Knerr, W. (2012). *Intimate partner violence [Fact Sheet].* Retrieved from https://apps.who.int/iris/bitstream/handle/10665/77432/WHO_RHR_12.36_eng.pdf?sequence=1

Glickman, C. (2012). *Escape the 'Act Like a Man' box.* Retrieved from https://goodmenproject.com/featured-content/megasahd-escape-the-act-like-a-man-box/

HeForShe.org. (2019). *Join the global movement.* Retrieved from www.heforshe.org/en

Heise, L., Ellsberg, M., & Gottmoeller, M. (1999). *Ending violence against women* (Population Reports, Series L, No. 11, pp. 1–43). Baltimore, MD: Population Information Program, The Johns Hopkins School of Public Health.

Heise, L., Ellsberg, M., & Gottmoeller, M. (2002). A global overview of gender-based violence. *International Journal of Gynecology and Obstetrics, 78*(S1). doi: 10.1016/S0020-7292(02)00038-3

Holland, K. J., Rabelo, V. C., Gustafson, A. M., Seabrook, R. C., & Cortina, L. M. (2016). Sexual harassment against men: Examining the roles of feminist activism, sexuality, and organizational context. *Psychology of Men & Masculinity, 17*(1), 17–29. doi: 10.1037/a0039151

Joyful Heart Foundation. (2019). *NO MORE excuses: The Male Survivors series.* Retrieved from www.joyfulheartfoundation.org/programs/education/no-more/psa-campaign/no-more-excuses-male-survivors-series

Kapur, A., & Muddell, K. (2016). *When no one calls it rape: Addressing sexual violence against men and boys in transitional contexts.* Retrieved from https://www.ictj.org/sites/default/files/ICTJ_Report_SexualViolenceMen_2016.pdf

ManKind Initiative. (2014). *#ViolenceIsViolence: Domestic abuse advert Mankind.* Retrieved from www.youtube.com/watch?v=u3PgH86OyEM

ManKind Initiative. (2019). *About us.* Retrieved from www.mankind.org.uk/about-us/

McLaughlin, H., Uggen, C., & Blackstone, A. (2012). Sexual harassment, workplace authority, and the paradox of power. *American Sociological Review, 77*(4), 625–647. doi: 10.1177/0003122412451728

MenCare & UN Women. (2014). *Men, masculinities & changing power.* Retrieved from http://menengage.org/wp-content/uploads/2015/03/MenEngage-brochure-for-CSW59_final2.pdf

National Resource Center on Domestic Violence (n.d.). *DVRN.* Retrieved from https://nrcdv.org/dvrn/

Office for National Statistics. (2019). *Domestic abuse in England and Wales overview: November 2019.* Retrieved from www.ons.gov.uk/peoplepopulationandcommunity/crimeandjustice/bulletins/domesticabuseinenglandandwalesoverview/november2019

Pan, A., Daley, S., Rivera, L. M., Williams, K., Lingle, D., & Reznik, V. (2006). Understanding the role of culture in domestic violence: The Ahimsa Project for Safe Families. *Journal of Immigrant and Minority Health, 8*(1), 35–43.

Pérez-Fuentes, G., Olfson, M., Villegas, L., Morcillo, C., Wang, S., & Blanco, C. (2013). Prevalence and correlates of child sexual abuse: A national study. *Comprehensive Psychiatry, 54*(1). doi: 10.1016/j.comppsych.2012.05.010

Pinheiro, P. S. (2006). *World report on violence against children.* Retrieved from https://resourcecentre. savethechildren.net/node/2999/pdf/2999.pdf

Skyhorse Publishing. (2019). *Breaking out of the "Man Box."* Retrieved from www.skyhorsepublishing. com/9781510701496/breaking-out-of-the-man-box/

Stermac, L., del Bove, G., & Addison, M. (2004). Stranger and acquaintance sexual assault of adult males. *Journal of Interpersonal Violence, 19*(8), 901–915.

Stewart, A. L. (2014). The Men's Project: A sexual assault prevention program targeting college men. *Psychology of Men & Masculinity, 15*(4), 481–485. http://dx.doi.org/10.1037/a0033947

United Nations. (2017). *Note to correspondents on sexual harassment.* Retrieved from https://www.un.org/ sg/en/content/sg/note-correspondents/2017-12-21/note-correspondents-sexual-harassment

UN Women. (2014). *Emma Watson: Gender equality is your issue too.* Retrieved from www.unwomen. org/en/news/stories/2014/9/emma-watson-gender-equality-is-your-issue-too

U.S. Department of Education. (2015). *Title IX and sex discrimination.* Retrieved from www2. ed.gov/about/offices/list/ocr/docs/tix_dis.html

U.S. Department of Justice. (n.d.). *Learn about hate crimes.* Retrieved from www.justice.gov/ hatecrimes/learn-about-hate-crimes

U.S. Department of Justice–Federal Bureau of Investigation. (2018). *Hate crime statistics.* Retrieved from https://ucr.fbi.gov/hate-crime/2017/topic-pages/victims.pdf

U.S. Equal Employment Opportunity Commission. (n.d.). *Charges alleging sexual harassment FY 2010–FY 2018.* Retrieved from www.eeoc.gov/eeoc/statistics/enforcement/sexual_harass-ment_new.cfm

Wells, J. (2015). *Why will no one fund male domestic abuse charities?* Retrieved from www.telegraph. co.uk/men/thinking-man/why-will-no-one-fund-male-domestic-abuse-charities/

World Health Organization. (2017). Retrieved from www.who.int/news-room/fact-sheets/detail/ violence-against-women

World Health Organization, United Nations Development Programme, & United Nations Office on Drugs and Crime. (2014). *New study highlights need to scale up violence prevention efforts globally* [Press Release]. Retrieved from www.who.int/violence_injury_prevention/violence/status_ report/2014/FINAL_GSRVP_2014_press_release_REV.pdf?ua=1

Part IV
Staying healthy

12 Alcohol, tobacco, and drugs

Adam E. Barry, Alex M. Russell, and Zachary A. Jackson

In this chapter, substance use will be presented from a men's health perspective. Emphasis is placed on alcohol as it is the most commonly used substance among men globally (World Health Organization [WHO], 2018a), and men are far more likely to drink excessively than women (Centers for Disease Control and Prevention [CDC], 2016a). In particular, we will provide a rationale for why alcohol consumption and associated consequences represent an important men's health issue. This chapter will also present important background on contemporary substance-use issues pertinent to young adults in college/university settings, such as marijuana use, vaping, and opioid abuse. Prior to beginning the chapter, it is important to first assess your personal biases and beliefs about alcohol, and substance use more broadly.

Personal assessment

Do you drink? Why or why not? What factors have impacted this decision?

Alcohol and the human body: A primer on how alcohol impacts you

Do you know the basic effects of alcohol? Simply put, alcohol acts as an irritant and sedative. Once consumed, alcohol initially begins to irritate internal tissues and subsequently sedates them as drinking continues. As alcohol sedates the brain, drinkers can have difficulty walking, slurred speech, blurred vision, delayed reaction times, and impaired memory. Alcohol affects the brain in the following order:

1. The first parts of the brain impacted by alcohol are the regions responsible for judgment, decision-making, reasoning, and inhibitions. Most of the consequences associated with drinking are directly associated with losses to reason and judgment (e.g., unprotected sex, sexual relations with a stranger, deciding to drive an automobile after drinking, violence, and aggression).
2. The second areas of the brain impacted by alcohol are those governing muscle control and bodily senses. Once impacted, your ability to walk, talk, and move in a coordinated manner will be reduced.
3. As drinking continues, it is possible that alcohol will sedate the portion of the brain associated with controlling vital functions (e.g., breathing). In other words, the

involuntary bodily functions governed by the brain (e.g., blood pressure, heart rate) can be impaired to a lethal level.

Alcohol consumption and associated consequences worldwide

For centuries, alcohol has been widely used across many different cultures. Attempts to ban drinking (i.e., prohibition) across history have failed, with the notable exception being persons or groups following religious rules/commands. For instance, alcohol use is prohibited in the Islamic faith. Intoxicating substances, with alcohol being the most common, have played a central role in every documented society. Among these societies and across cultures, alcohol has been uniformly used to note life transitions, celebrate milestones, and has been embedded in customs and rituals (Social Issues Research Centre, 1998). In modern society, alcohol use is often commonly accepted as a part of the social environment and considered culturally routine among many.

Approximately 2.3 billion people across the world are classified as current drinkers, with more than half of the population in America and Europe consuming alcohol (WHO, 2018c). It isn't surprising, therefore, if someone were to ask "do you want to grab a drink?," you would probably assume an alcoholic drink was implied. Because alcohol is essentially everywhere – whether that be as part of your social landscape, in the contemporary art and media you interact with, or in the music, movies, television, and advertising you are exposed to – it can be easy to overlook the negative health and social ramifications associated with drinking.

The highest levels of alcohol per capita consumption are in the World Health Organization's European Region. This region includes, but is not limited to, countries such as France, Greece, Poland, Romania, the Russian Federation, and Ukraine. The range of average alcohol consumption per day among current drinkers is as high as 40 grams per day (g/day) of pure alcohol (African region) to as low as 26.3 g/day (South-east Asia) (WHO, 2018b). Approximately one-fourth of all alcohol consumed worldwide is considered unrecorded alcohol (WHO, 2018b). Unrecorded alcohol is illegally produced, distributed, and sold outside governmentally controlled and regulated channels (e.g., alcohol such as homebrew or moonshine that a person or small group creates). Compared to persons residing in industrialized countries, a substantially higher proportion of people in lower and middle-income countries consume unrecorded alcohol. Almost half of the recorded alcohol consumed worldwide is in the form of spirits, followed by beer (34%) and wine (12%) (WHO, 2018b).

Globally, alcohol use contributes to 3 million deaths annually, representing just over 5% of the world's total deaths (WHO, 2018b). Among those between the ages of 20 and 39, roughly 14% of deaths are associated with alcohol consumption – the leading cause of premature death among this population (WHO, 2018b). More than one out of every four persons worldwide between the ages of 15 and 19 years old are current drinkers, amounting to approximately 155 million adolescents (WHO, 2018c). Prevalence rates of current drinking among 15–19 year olds is highest in the European region (WHO, 2018b). This is particularly troubling given the brain continues to develop up until around the age of 25, making the adolescent brain particularly susceptible to the detrimental effects of alcohol. Drinking is directly associated with over 200 different diseases and injuries, including various forms of cancer, cardiovascular disease, and other noncommunicable diseases (American Cancer Society, 2017; WHO, 2018a). Traffic collisions, violence, and suicides connected with alcohol consumption contribute to a widespread number of injuries and deaths, especially among younger age groups (WHO, 2018a). Similarly, harmful alcohol use has been identified as a contributing factor to numerous mental and behavioral disorders (WHO, 2018a). Harmful alcohol use also creates a negative impact on the economy and society at large (WHO, 2018a). For example, the cost of excessive alcohol use in the United States for a single year was approximated to be $249 billion (CDC, 2018). Globally, an estimated 237 million men have an alcohol-use disorder (AUD), with the highest prevalence of AUD among persons in the European region and the region of the Americas, a region including North-, Central-, and Southern-America countries (WHO, 2018b). Alcohol-attributable disease burden is highest in low-income and lower-middle-income countries, compared to upper-middle-income and high-income countries (WHO, 2018b). Thus, reducing the health, societal, and economic burden associated with alcohol use represents an important global public health goal.

In his own words

Anonymous

As a Black college student, I expected to drink, of course, because that is what college students do. I drank to feel good, make friends, celebrate acing an exam, or to forget about bombing an exam. However, when college life was no longer a novelty, drinking became a masculine guise to mask vulnerability for my friends and me. Many of my friends and I were socialized to believe manhood means bearing through and surviving struggles without complaining or showing emotion. But there were many times the stressors of life became too much to bear alone. In these moments, when we drank together, expressing our feelings and sharing our emotions became socially acceptable because it was done over alcohol. These moments were potentially damaging because sometimes we drank more than we should have. Yet, they were also cathartic and bonded us together. They allowed us to release the pressures of our situations, which was invaluable, given none of us, at that time, sought mental health services.

If alcohol consumption results in so much death and disability, and there are so many costs associated with drinking, why do people drink? This is an incredibly difficult question to answer, as the reasons are different for each person, and differ across the life-span depending on social and environmental factors/pressures. Some drinkers may use alcohol as a "social lubricant," alleviating their social anxiety and reducing inhibitions. Others may enjoy alcohol as a form of stress relief or way to wind down after a long day. Others may enjoy the camaraderie and social bonding that comes with drinking. Theoretical frameworks trying to understand the varied reasons and factors impacting alcohol use recognize the complexity of this issue and typically adopt a social-ecological framework, which contends human health and behavior of an individual is nested within broader, more macro-level influences. Specifically, the behavior of individuals is influenced by their personal beliefs and cognitions, as well as their immediate social and physical environments (e.g., school, home, work). These smaller social and physical environments are also nested within larger social and political environments (i.e., state/province, country) which can also influence behavior through broader rules, regulations, and policies (Bronfenbrenner, 1994). While the factors influencing one's drinking are varied and individualistic, researchers have noted four primary personal motivations for drinking alcohol (Kuntsche, Knibbe, Gmel, & Engels, 2006):

1. *enhancement*: drinking to enhance mood (e.g., feel better);
2. *social*: drinking to be social in social settings (e.g., parties, dinners);
3. *conformity*: drinking to "fit in," or consuming alcohol because others around you are drinking;
4. *coping*: drinking as a form of medicating; drinking to forget or deal with problems.

Coping motives, in particular, have demonstrated a direct link to unique alcohol-related problems over time. Drinking to cope is strongly correlated with one's perceived stress levels (Abbey, Smith, & Scott, 1993). Persons whose drinking is driven by a desire to alleviate negative emotions or cognition are at increased risk for problematic alcohol-related outcomes (Merrell, Wardell, & Read, 2014).

Personal assessment

What are some of the societal and/or environmental forces that affect your substance-use behaviors?

Societal influences on drinking

While each of us wants to believe that we alone make our own decisions and choices, there are many external factors and societal forces that impact our thoughts, beliefs, and behaviors. Alcohol advertising, in particular, has demonstrated a strong association with drinking behaviors. Specifically, it has been well established that traditional media alcohol advertising, such as print magazines and televised commercials and programs, negatively impacts the age at which one first tries alcohol and increases overall drinking quantity among those who already consume alcohol (Anderson, De Bruijn, Angus, Gordon, & Hastings, 2009; Smith & Foxcroft, 2009). Alcohol commercials have been shown to particularly affect younger adolescents' propensity to consume alcohol (Grenard, Dent, & Stacy, 2013). The alcohol industry intentionally employs targeted marketing strategies aimed at certain demographic groups (i.e., African American), age groups (i.e., youth), and gender (i.e., men). Drinkers, especially young male drinkers, are much more likely to be exposed to alcohol advertising. Men, and particularly young men, see more alcohol advertisements of all types than females. For instance, men see more than two times the number of beer advertisements that women do (Lillard, Molloy, & Zan, 2018). Examinations of a decade's worth of beer advertisements airing across national markets highlighted the most common advertisement violations included linking beer drinking with social success and utilizing content that would clearly be appealing to persons younger than 21 years of age (Babor, Xuan, Damon, & Noel, 2013). In-depth investigations of almost 600 unique television alcohol advertisements from the top 20 U.S. beer and spirit brands identified five distinct content categories: partying, quality, sports, manliness, and relaxation. Party-related content, which included ads centered on love, sex, and socialization, comprised almost half (42%) of all these advertisements (Morgenstern et al., 2015). Targeted marketing strategies, such as these, lead to individuals developing positive beliefs about drinking, and expanding the environments in which they believe alcohol use is socially acceptable (Hastings, Anderson, Cooke, & Gordon, 2005).

Personal assessment

Do you think men are especially prone to drink? What about men, or our societal views of a man, make them more likely to consume alcohol?

Who drinks more? Examining alcohol consumption across sexes

As previously outlined, it is important to note that there are a wide variety of factors affecting alcohol consumption and alcohol-related harm, ranging from individual-based factors to social/environmental factors. Moreover, these factors are also intertwined with the actual individual consumption behaviors, such as the pattern in which certain quantities are consumed. That said, men and women, on average, tend to partake in different levels and patterns of alcohol consumption. For instance, male drinkers worldwide consume almost three times as much alcohol as female drinkers (WHO, 2018a; 2018b). American men are almost two times more likely to binge drink than American females (CDC, 2016a). As such, men tend to experience more health-related consequences associated with their drinking. Globally, approximately 8% of deaths among men can be attributed to alcohol, while only 3% of deaths among women are alcohol-attributable (WHO, 2018a). Of the 3 million alcohol-attributable deaths in 2016, more than three out of four of these deaths were among men (WHO, 2018b). Moreover, approximately 237 million men suffer from AUDs compared to 46 million women (WHO, 2018b). Thus, it is quite clear that alcohol use represents an important men's health issue given men are disproportionately affected by drinking compared to their female peers.

Alcohol-related biological differences between men and women

Due to biological differences, men absorb and process alcohol differently than women, making them less susceptible to intoxication. Simply put, because of several factors, men will become intoxicated slower than their female counterparts. These reasons include:

- Men have higher amounts, and more active, alcohol dehydrogenase (ADH) in their bodies compared to women. ADH is the enzyme that breaks down (i.e., metabolizes) alcohol. Men metabolize alcohol more efficiently. Therefore, men will absorb less alcohol into their bloodstreams compared to females – even when drinking the same quantity.
- Alcohol is water soluble and dissipates into the body's water. Fat (adipose) tissue essentially retains alcohol. In other words, alcohol will not enter fatty tissue, but rather resides in water. Overall, men (a) *generally* have higher total body water quantities than women, and (b) *generally* have a lower body fat percentage than females. This means that men will reach a lower blood alcohol concentration (BAC) if they consume the same amount of alcohol at a similar rate as a similarly sized female.

- Males, on average, have larger body masses compared to females. Larger persons will have a lower BAC, compared to another person of the same gender who weighs less, even if they consume the same amount of alcohol across the same time-period. Consider the following analogy: if you pour the same amount of sugar into an eight-ounce glass of tea and a one-gallon pitcher of tea, which would be sweeter? Obviously, the smaller glass would be much sweeter tea than the gallon pitcher. Even though the sugar content is the same in both containers, it is more concentrated in the smaller container.

Though men process alcohol more efficiently than women, it begs the question: "Why do they experience disproportionately more negative effects of drinking than females?"

Alcohol-related issues specific to men

Because men are more likely to partake in hazardous drinking than females, men are at a higher risk for short- and long-term health-related consequences associated with their drinking (e.g., aggression and violence, hospitalizations, alcohol-related deaths, suicides) (CDC, 2016a). Additionally, there are important alcohol-related issues specific to men. Though a man may feel more confident after a drink or two, alcohol will not help his sexual performance. Given alcohol is a central nervous system depressant, alcohol consumption can negatively interfere with men being able to achieve, and maintain, an erection (Grover, Mattoo, Pendharkar, & Kandappan, 2014). Drinking can also lead to reductions in testosterone, which can result in reduced sperm count and quality, as well as loss of your sexual desire (i.e., libido) (Emanuele & Emanuele, 1998).

While alcohol represents "empty calories," which by their very nature could lead to increased body mass, drinking alcohol actually results in your body burning less fat – removing residual alcohol in your body takes precedence over normal bodily functions, such as burning fat and absorbing nutrients (Sharma, 2015). Excessive alcohol consumption can also intensify skin conditions, such as rosacea, resulting in inflammation, and a reddening of the face (Spoendlin, Voegel, Jick, & Meir, 2012).

Compared to women, men report more deaths and nonfatal hospitalizations due to excessive alcohol use. Specifically, men who consume excessive quantities of alcohol are more likely to die of liver cancer, a stroke, alcoholic liver disease, and alcohol-associated heart disease (Stahre & Simon, 2010).

Simply put, the health consequences associated with alcohol use among men are numerous.

Alcohol use among men across the lifespan

In general, overall alcohol consumption declines with age. However, for a small proportion of demographic groups, such as the affluent, highly educated, and men, drinking increases with age (Bobo, Greek, Klepinger, & Herting, 2013). This is concerning for that small minority of people because as people age, they become more vulnerable to the physiologic effects of alcohol. Specifically, as one ages, the enzymes that metabolize alcohol and other substances become less efficient (Ferreira & Weems, 2008; Gargiulo et al., 2013). Additionally, as people become older, the likelihood that they will take medication increases. Thus, older adults who consume alcohol are more likely to be taking alcohol-interactive medications (Breslow, Dong, & White, 2015).

Substance use in college settings

For both men and women, college is a time when they may experiment with alcohol and other drugs. Annually, more than 1,800 college students die as a result of unintentional injuries (Hingson, Zha, & Weitzman, 2009), almost 700,000 are assaulted by another student who has been drinking alcohol (Hingson, Heeren, Winter, & Wechsler, 2005), and about one of every four students report academic consequences due to drinking (Kerr, Patterson, Koenen, & Greenfield, 2008). Though alcohol use is most common among college students, the National Institute on Drug Abuse contends marijuana, vaping, and prescription drug misuse have been steadily increasing among college-aged adults (National Institute on Drug Abuse [NIDA], 2017).

Cannabis (a general term encompassing many different psychoactive variations of the Cannabis sativa plant) is the most abused and trafficked illicit drug in the world (WHO, 2019a). Just under 3% of the global population consume cannabis, representing approximately 147 million individuals. Over the past several decades, the most rapid increases in cannabis use and abuse have occurred in Australia, North America, and Western Europe. In particular, cannabis use is most closely linked to youth and young adults (WHO, 2019a).

Marijuana typically refers to the cannabis leaves and/or other cannabis plant materials. Marijuana use among college students has continued to increase, reaching its highest levels in the past 30 years. Nearly 40% of college students between the ages of 19 and 22 report marijuana use at least once in the past year, while 13% report daily marijuana use (Schulenberg et al., 2018). The increasing use of marijuana has been attributed to declines in the perceived risks and harm of marijuana use (Schulenberg et al., 2018). Additionally, across the United States, more states are considering legalizing recreational marijuana use, which may impact a person's belief that marijuana is safe. That said, even if a state has legalized marijuana there are still inherent risks in using marijuana and important legal context to remember. For instance, marijuana's negative effects on a person's learning, attention, and memory can take days after the initial high to wear off (Tapert, Schweinsburg, & Brown, 2008). Students who smoke marijuana have worse educational outcomes than their non-smoking peers (Macleod et al., 2004). If a college or university in the United States is in a legalized state, the institution is still required to abide by the federal Safe and Drug-Free Schools and Communities Act. Essentially, this means that federal (country-wide) policies trump state policies. Thus, all institutions of higher education must maintain policies prohibiting marijuana possession, use, or distribution even if the state they reside in has legalized marijuana use. Furthermore, this means that even persons with a prescription would be prohibited from storing or using their medical marijuana on campus.

E-cigarettes are battery-operated devices that heat up a liquid blend of nicotine, flavorings, and other chemicals, which results in an aerosol that is inhaled by the user. The aerosol produced by vaping devices may contain cancer-causing agents, heavy metals (e.g., tin, nickel, lead), ultra-fine particles that can be inhaled deep into the lungs, as well as flavorings linked with lung disease (U.S. Department of Health and Human Services [USHHS], 2016). There is limited research examining the long-term safety and health effects associated with vaping. That said, the research available points to vaping being a serious public health issue. Just like combustible cigarettes, e-cigarettes contain highly addictive nicotine, which is detrimental to brain development and can increase the risk for addiction to other drugs (USHHS, 2016). Additionally, defective e-cigarette batteries can explode or cause fires, resulting in serious injury. There have also been reports of children and adults being poisoned by swallowing, breathing, or absorbing e-cigarette liquid (CDC, 2019).

Though frequently marketed by the tobacco industry as a "quit smoking aid," there is much debate regarding the usefulness of vaping to reduce cigarette use. The Food and Drug Administration (FDA) has not approved e-cigarettes as a quit smoking aid. Moreover, there is research suggesting that people who attempted to quit smoking cigarettes by vaping, instead continue to use both cigarettes and e-cigarettes (CDC, 2016b). The vast majority of colleges and universities that have enacted smoke-free campus policies specifically prohibit the use of e-cigarettes as well (Wang et al., 2018). The World Health Organization has advocated that all central and local governments adopt regulations that designate any indoor smoke-free areas also be vape-free areas, an approach already being implemented by more than 25 countries (Wilson, Hoek, Thomson, & Edwards, 2017).

Opioids are psychoactive substances derived from the opium poppy plant (e.g., heroin) or synthetically produced opioids using the same chemical structure (e.g., fentanyl). Opioids (e.g., oxycodone, codeine, and hydrocodone) are commonly used for pain management, but require a doctor's prescription to be consumed legally. Worldwide, approximately 34 million people used opioids and 19 million used opiates in the past year. It is estimated that 27 million people suffer from opioid use disorders, with the majority of these dependent users consuming illegally developed and obtained heroin; yet, increasing number of users are illegally abusing prescription opioids. Because opioids affect the region of the brain that controls breathing, high doses can negatively impact respiration and ultimately lead to death. Opioids represent a very large proportion of the fatal drug overdoses occurring each year (WHO, 2019b).

Prescription stimulant medications, such as Adderall or Ritalin, are sometimes abused as "study drugs" to increase concentration and alertness for the purpose of studying and pulling "all-nighters." It is important to note that both purchasing and/or consuming prescription medications without a valid doctor's prescription, and selling your own personal prescribed medication to others, is illegal. Illegally using or distributing prescription drugs can have far reaching implications, ranging from legal (i.e., police citations, arrests) to academic (i.e., student conduct and academic integrity violations, dismissal) (NIDA, 2018).

Finally, any perceived benefit from study drugs can actually be achieved via a healthy lifestyle. Exercising can help recover from mental fatigue associated with studying, aid in coping with stress from academic deadlines/assessments, and also lead to increased energy and improved blood flow. Focused breathing exercises and meditation can also help you decompress and improve focus. Eating a healthy, well-rounded diet can also have a positive impact on your energy levels and focus. Lack of quality sleep time can result in worse cognitive functioning, inability to focus, and difficulty completing mental tasks. Thus, taking good care of yourself − through regular intentional exercise, a balanced diet, and proper sleep − will have a better impact on your academics than study drugs.

Being substance use free in college

While excessive alcohol use does happen in college settings, it is important to note that large proportions of college students (four out of every ten) report not consuming alcohol in the past 30 days (Substance Abuse and Mental Health Services [SAMHSA], 2015a). Moreover, almost nine out of every ten college students report they do not drink heavily (i.e., consuming five or more drinks (males) or four or more drinks (females) within a couple hours more than once a week) (SAMHSA, 2015b).

In his own words

Anonymous

When I entered into the college environment, I had experimented with alcohol and drugs. However, my "partying" quickly became out of control my freshman year. For the first time I was on my own away from my parents. I perceived that all my peers, or at least the cool ones, were partying and using drugs/alcohol. This desire to fit in was what initially fueled my alcohol and drug use, but eventually I became addicted and was using alcohol and drugs daily to cope with life and to feel good. I began skipping classes and making terrible grades, spending all of my money on alcohol and drugs, and eventually was arrested for possession of illegal drugs. My entire life turned upside down, and I had to seek treatment for my addiction. In doing so, I took a semester off from school and lived in a sober living facility. When I eventually returned to school, I discovered my university had a collegiate recovery community. This community consisted of a group of my student peers who were also seeking recovery from substance and/or behavioral addiction/s. The recovery community was vital to my recovery, academics, and overall college experience. We had access to 12-step meetings on campus and academic counseling, and we hosted social activities like sober tailgating and hiking trips. Like most of my peers in the recovery community, I thrived in my final years of college and had a great experience!

Many universities in the United States offer amenities to help foster a college experience that is not focused on alcohol or other drugs. This could include substance-free dorms where students live with others interested in a college experience free of alcohol and drug use. Colleges and universities are also providing alcohol-free social, extra-curricular, and recreational options and events to help provide students with social opportunities free of substance use. In order to serve the growing number of college students in recovery from an addiction, some colleges have fostered the development of Collegiate Recovery Communities (CRCs). CRCs provide recovery support services and promote academic growth, offering a variety of services to recovering students, including but not limited to 12-step meetings, peer social support, academic support, sober recreational activities, and sober living arrangements. CRCs also offer dedicated support staff and physical space for students to gather, meet, and socialize safely and soberly (Cleveland, Harris, Baker, Herbert, & Dean, 2007; Laudet, Harris, Kimball, Winters, & Moberg, 2014).

Learning more about substance use from a male perspective

Developed as a public health campaign in the United Kingdom, Dry January, has emerged as a cultural phenomenon increasing people's awareness of their alcohol consumption behaviors. Essentially, Dry January is a New Year's resolution where someone commits to not drinking alcohol during the entire month of January. Millions of people annually engage in this event – check out #DryJanuary on social media.

As you reflect on your own relationship with alcohol, and perhaps contemplate abstaining for 31 days next January, check out the following books:

- *The Unexpected Joys of Being Sober: Discovering a Happy, Healthy, Wealthy Alcohol-Free Life.* By Catherine Gray (2017).
- *Alcohol is SH!T: How to Ditch the Booze, Re-ignite Your Life, and Recover the Person you Were Always Meant to Be.* By Paul Churchill (2019).

The following movies show the impact alcohol can have on our relationships with others:

- *Smashed* (2012)
- *Crazy Heart* (2009)

Advancing men's health and substance-use behaviors

One of the most crucial ways to help men improve public health and their own quality of life is to have them engage in self-reflection about their drinking and substance use. Often, we simply get into routines without cognitively thinking about how our behaviors may be negatively impacting our health. Read the books and watch the movies outlined in this chapter. Have you experienced similar consequences as those discussed and depicted because of your personal substance-use behaviors? At the very least, purposefully reflect on your own behaviors and whether they align with the goals and desires you have for your personal and professional life. There are a litany of tools and resources online to help you in this process. For instance, the National Institute of Health hosts a "Rethinking Drinking" website (www.rethinkingdrinking.niaaa.nih.gov/) that would be a great starting point, as it has features that allow you to check your drinking pattern and compare and contrast your behaviors to standardized guidelines. As an adult male, there are many resources at your disposal should you, or those around you, have concerns about your substance-use behaviors. The groups outlined below all have great resources and the social support necessary to help you achieve your healthiest, best self.

Did you know?

Al-Anon provides support to "people, just like you, who are worried about someone with a drinking problem" (n.d., para. 1).

Alcoholics Anonymous (AA) is an international organization for "anyone who wants to do something about his or her drinking problem" (2019, para. 1). To find meetings in the United States or Canada, visit www.aa.org. To find meetings in Europe or online, visit https://alcoholics-anonymous.eu/ or download the Meeting Finder app.

Narcotics Anonymous (NA) is a worldwide organization that is open to anyone using any drug or substance who wants to stop using. NA has over 70,000 meetings that are held in more than 140 countries (Narcotics Anonymous, 2018).

References

Abbey, A., Smith, M. J., & Scott, R. O. (1993). The relationship between reasons for drinking alcohol and alcohol consumption: An interactional approach. *Addictive Behaviors, 18*(6), 659–670.

Al-anon. (n.d.). *Who are al-anon members?* Retrieved from https://al-anon.org/

Alcoholics Anonymous. (2019). *What is A.A.?* Retrieved from www.aa.org/pages/en_US/what-is-aa

American Cancer Society. (2017). *Alcohol Use and Cancer.* Atlanta, GA: ACS.

Anderson, P., De Bruijn, A., Angus, K., Gordon, R., & Hastings, G. (2009). Impact of alcohol advertising and media exposure on adolescent alcohol use: A systematic review of longitudinal studies. *Alcohol and Alcoholism, 44*(3), 229–243.

Babor, T. F., Xuan, Z., Damon, D., & Noel, J. (2013). An empirical evaluation of the US Beer Institute's self-regulation code governing the content in beer advertising. *American Journal of Public Health, 103*(10), 45–51.

Bobo, J. K., Greek, A. A., Klepinger, D. H., & Herting, J. R. (2013). Predicting 10-year alcohol use trajectories among men age 50 years and older. *American Journal of Geriatric Psychiatry, 21*(2), 204–213.

Breslow, R. A., Dong, C., & White, A. (2015). Prevalence of alcohol-interactive prescription medication use among current drinkers: United States, 1999 to 2010. *Alcoholism: Clinical & Experimental Research, 39*(2), 371–379.

Bronfenbrenner, U. (1994). *International Encyclopedia of Education, 2nd ed.* Oxford, UK: Elsevier. Ecological models of human development, pp. 1643–1647.

Centers for Disease Control and Prevention. (2016a). *Alcohol.* Retrieved from www.cdc.gov/alcohol/fact-sheets/mens-health.htm

Centers for Disease Control and Prevention. (2016b). QuickStats: Cigarette smoking status among current adult e-cigarette users, by age group—National Health Interview Survey, United States, 2015. *MMWR, 65,* 1177.

Centers for Disease Control and Prevention. (2018). *Excessive drinking is draining the U.S. economy.* Retrieved from www.cdc.gov/features/costsofdrinking/index.html

Centers for Disease Control and Prevention. (2019). *About electronic cigarettes (E-cigarettes).* Retrieved from www.cdc.gov/tobacco/basic_information/e-cigarettes/about-e-cigarettes.html

Cleveland, H. H., Harris, K. S., Baker, A. K., Herbert, R., & Dean, L. R. (2007). Characteristics of a collegiate recovery community: Maintaining recovery in an abstinence-hostile environment. *Journal of Substance Abuse Treatment, 33*(1), 13–23. https://doi.org/10.1016/j.jsat.2006.11.005

Emanuele, M. A., & Emanuele, N. V. (1998). Alcohol's effects on male reproduction. *Alcohol Research and Health, 22*(3), 195–201.

Ferreira, M. P., & Weems, M. K. (2008). Alcohol consumption by aging adults in the United States: Health benefits and detriments. *Journal of the American Dietetic Association, 108*(10), 1668–1676.

Gargiulo, G., Testa, G., Cacciatore, F., Mazzella, F., Galizia, G., Della-Morte, D., ... Abete, P. (2013). Moderate alcohol consumption predicts long-term mortality in elderly subjects with chronic heart failure. *Journal of Nutrition, Health, & Aging, 17*(5), 480–485.

Grenard, J. L., Dent, C. W., Stacy, A. W. (2013). Exposure to alcohol advertisements and teenage alcohol-related problems. *Pediatrics,* 131(2), e369–e379.

Grover, S., Mattoo, S. K., Pendharkar, S., & Kandappan, V. (2014). Sexual dysfunction in patients with alcohol and opioid dependence. *Indian Journal of Psychological Medicine, 36*(4), 355–365.

Hastings, G., Anderson, S., Cooke, E., Gordon, R. (2005). Alcohol marketing and young people's drinking: A review of the research. *Journal of Public Health Policy, 26*(3), 296–311.

Hingson, R., Heeren, T., Winter, M., & Wechsler, H. (2005). Magnitude of alcohol-related mortality and morbidity among US college students ages 18–24: Changes from 1998 to 2001. *Annual Review of Public Health, 26,* 259–279.

Hingson, R. W., Zha, W., & Weitzman, E. R. (2009). Magnitude of and trends in alcohol-related mortality and morbidity among US college students ages 18–24, 1998–2005. *Journal of Studies on Alcohol and Drugs, Supplement*, (16), 12–20.

Kerr, W. C., Patterson, D., Koenen, M. A., & Greenfield, T. K. (2008). Alcohol content variation of bar and restaurant drinks in northern California. *Alcoholism: Clinical & Experimental Research*, *32*(9), 1623–1629.

Kuntsche, E., Knibbe, R., Gmel, G., & Engels, R. (2006). Replication and validation of the Drinking Motive Questionnaire Revised (DMQ-R, Cooper, 1994) among adolescents in Switzerland. *European Addiction Research*, *12*(3), 161–168.

Laudet, A., Harris, K., Kimball, T., Winters, K. C., & Moberg, D. P. (2014). Collegiate recovery communities programs: What do we know and what do we need to know? *Journal of Social Work Practice in the Addictions*, *14*, 84–100.

Lillard, D. R., Molloy, E., & Zan, H. (2018). Television and magazine alcohol advertising: Exposure and trends by sex and age. *Journal of Studies on Alcohol and Drugs*, *79*(6), 881–892.

Macleod, J., Oakes, R., Copello, A., Crome, I., Egger, M., Hickman, M., … & Smith, G. D. (2004). Psychological and social sequelae of cannabis and other illicit drug use by young people: A systematic review of longitudinal, general population studies. *The Lancet*, *363*(9421), 1579–1588.

Merrell, J. Æ., Wardell, J. D., & Read, J. P. (2014). Drinking motives in the prospective prediction of unique alcohol-related consequences in college students. *Journal of Studies on Alcohol and Drugs*, *75*(1), 93–102.

Morgenstern, M., Schoeppe, F., Campbell, J., Braam, M. W., Stoolmiller, M., & Sargent, J. D. (2015). Content themes of alcohol advertising in U.S. television: Latent class analysis. *Alcohol: Clinical & Experimental Research*, *39*(9), 1766–1774.

Narcotics Anonymous. (2018). *Information about NA*. Retrieved from www.na.org/admin/include/spaw2/uploads/pdf/pr/Info_about_NA_2016.pdf

National Institute on Drug Abuse. (2017). *Drug & alcohol use in college-age adults in 2017*. Retrieved from www.drugabuse.gov/related-topics/trends-statistics/infographics/drug-alcohol-use-in-college-age-adults-in-2017

National Institute on Drug Abuse. (2018). *Prescription stimulants*. Retrieved from www.drugabuse.gov/publications/drugfacts/prescription-stimulants

Schulenberg, J. E., Johnston, L. D., O'Malley, P. M., Bachman, J. G., Miech, R. A., & Patrick, M. E. (2018). *Monitoring the Future national survey results on drug use, 1975–2017: Volume II, College students and adults ages 19–55*. Ann Arbor: Institute for Social Research, The University of Michigan. Available at http://monitoringthefuture.org/pubs.html#monographs

Sharma, L. (2015). Effects of alcohol on mental and physical health of a sports person. *International Journal of Physical Education, Sports and Health*, *1*(4), 92–94.

Smith, L. A., & Foxcroft, D. R. (2009). The effect of alcohol advertising, marketing and portrayal on drinking behaviour in young people: Systematic review of prospective cohort studies. *BMC Public Health*, *9*(51).

Social Issues Research Centre. (1998). *Social and cultural aspects of drinking: A report to the European Commission*. Oxford, UK.

Spoendlin, J., Voegel, J., Jick, S., & Meier, C. (2012). A study on the epidemiology of rosacea in the U.K. *British Journal of Dermatology*, *167*(3), 598–605.

Stahre, M., & Simon, M. (2010). Alcohol-related deaths and hospitalizations by race, gender, and age in California. *The Open Epidemiology Journal*, *3*, 3–15.

Substance Abuse and Mental Health Services Administration. (2015a). *2015 national survey on drug use and health (NSDUH). Table 2.6B – Tobacco product and alcohol use in lifetime, past year, and past month among persons aged 18 or older: Percentages, 2014 and 2015*. Retrieved from www.samhsa.gov/data/sites/default/files/NSDUH-DetTabs-2015/NSDUH-DetTabs-2015/NSDUH-DetTabs-2015.htm#tab2-6b.

Substance Abuse and Mental Health Services Administration. (2015b). *2015 national survey on drug use and health (NSDUH). Table 6.84B – Tobacco product and alcohol use in past month among persons aged 18 to 22, by college enrollment status: Percentages, 2014 and 2015.* Retrieved from www.samhsa.gov/data/sites/default/files/NSDUH-DetTabs-2015/NSDUH-DetTabs-2015/NSDUH-DetTabs-2015.htm#tab6-84b

Tapert, S. F., Schweinsburg, A. D., & Brown, S. A. (2008). The influence of marijuana use on neurocognitive functioning in adolescents. *Current Drug Abuse Reviews, 1*(1), 99–111.

U.S. Department of Health and Human Services. (2016). *E-cigarette use among youth and young adults: A report of the Surgeon General.* Atlanta, GA: US Department of Health and Human Services, CDC.

Wang, T. W., Tynan, M. A., Hallett, C., Walpert, L., Hopkins, M., Konter, D., & King, B. A. (2018). Smoke-free and tobacco-free policies in colleges and universities: United States and territories, 2017. *Morbidity and Mortality Weekly Report, 67*(24), 686–689.

Wilson, N., Hoek, J., Thomson, G., & Edwards, R. (2017). Should e-cigarette use be included in indoor smoking bans? *Bulletin of the World Health Organization, 95*, 540–541.

World Health Organization. (2018a). *Alcohol.* Retrieved from www.who.int/news-room/fact-sheets/detail/alcohol

World Health Organization. (2018b). *Global status report on alcohol and health 2018.* Retrieved from www.who.int/substance_abuse/publications/global_alcohol_report/msbgsruprofiles.pdf

World Health Organization. (2018c). *Harmful use of alcohol kills more than 3 million people each year, most of them men.* Retrieved from www.who.int/news-room/detail/21-09-2018-harmful-use-of-alcohol-kills-more-than-3-million-people-each-year--most-of-them-men

World Health Organization. (2019a). *Cannabis: Facts and figures.* Retrieved from www.who.int/substance_abuse/facts/cannabis/en/

World Health Organization. (2019b). *Information sheet on opioid overdose.* Retrieved from www.who.int/substance_abuse/information-sheet/en/

13 Nutrition

Katie Potestio

Global perspective

Food provides the energy and nutrients necessary for growth and survival of every human being. Nutrition science examines the relationship between food and health and is based on the science of metabolism and biochemistry. According to the World Health Organization ([WHO] 2019b), nutrition is the intake of food, considered in relation to the body's dietary needs. Good nutrition is having an adequate and well-balanced diet. Together, good nutrition and regular physical activity are key influencers of health outcomes and longevity for people around the globe. The foundation of a healthy diet is similar across the world, even though food choices, flavors, and cultures vary drastically. Many countries develop their own national guidelines for nutrition, yet all the guidelines emphasize foods including fruits, vegetables, whole grains, and lean (low-fat) protein for good nutrition.

National guidelines for diet planning in the United States

Many countries publish dietary guidelines and food guides to translate the science of healthy eating into practical food patterns. In the United States, the U.S. Departments of Health and Human Services (HHS) and Agriculture (USDA) jointly publish a report containing nutritional and dietary information and guidelines for the general American public. The report is called the *Dietary Guidelines for Americans* and provides guidance for choosing a healthy diet and focuses on preventing the most common diet-related chronic diseases in the United States (U.S. Department of Health and Human Services and U.S. Department of Agriculture [HHS/USDA], 2015). The recommendations from the *Dietary Guidelines* are intended for Americans of all ages – children, adolescents, adults, and older adults. A new edition is published every five years to reflect the current scientific and medical knowledge. The *Dietary Guidelines* are used by health professionals and policymakers in developing federal food, nutrition, and health policies and programs. The relationship between diet and physical activity contributes to managing body weight so, beginning in 2008, HHS also began publishing *Physical Activity Guidelines for Americans* to help promote health and reduce the risk of chronic disease (HHS, 2018). To learn more, visit: health.gov/dietaryguidelines.

Poor nutrition, either not meeting or exceeding the body's dietary needs, increases the risk of disease by reducing immunity, impairing physical and mental development, and leading to metabolic/physiological changes such as elevated blood pressure, overweight/obesity, blood glucose, and cholesterol (WHO, 2019b). These changes, in turn, can cause chronic diseases, such as heart disease, cancer, and diabetes, and premature death. WHO

(2019a) projects that 80% of premature heart disease, stroke, and diabetes can be prevented with lifestyle changes such as healthier food choices.

The cost of poor nutrition can harm individuals, institutions, economies, and even the peace and stability of nations (Development Initiatives, 2018). Similarly, the benefits of good nutrition can have a ripple effect that impacts not only individuals, but entire populations and the environment (Development Initiatives, 2018).

In his own words

Meet Issa

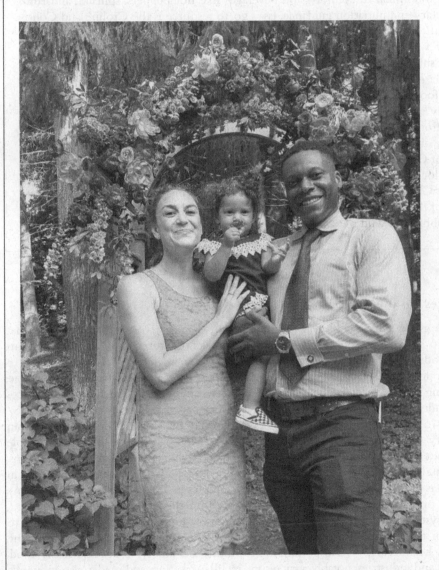

Figure 13.1 Issa with his family at his U.S. Citizenship Naturalization Ceremony.
Source: Printed with permission.

Issa is a 30-year-old man living in Maryland with his partner and daughter. He proudly hails from Trinidad and Tobago. He became a U.S. Citizen in 2018, a year after his daughter was born. He works as a Customer Support Database Administrator. Issa also has ulcerative colitis, a chronic disease of the large intestine that causes long-lasting inflammation and sores in the digestive tract. When he was diagnosed at age 22, it transformed the way he ate. Now this chronic disease remains one of the main factors that influences what he eats. As with other diseases of the digestive tract, ulcerative colitis often requires people to make significant dietary changes. Issa found that he felt much better when he followed the recommended dietary pattern and avoided trigger foods (i.e. foods that cause him to feel abdominal discomfort) and beverages like hot peppers, spinach, and rum. For dietary and nutrition guidance, Issa's go-to resource is the Crohn's and Colitis Foundation (www.crohnscolitisfoundation.org) and the Foundation's online community where he can participate in discussion boards, share and hear personal stories, submit questions.

While growing up in Trinidad and Tobago, Issa's diet consisted mainly of traditional foods eaten at home with his family. He ate breakfast every day before school, typically eggs and bread with peanut butter or honey. For lunch, he would come home from school to enjoy a three-course meal with his family over some of his favorite dishes, such as curry and chana (dishes originating in India), and callaloo (a staple of Creole cooking). Trinidad and Tobago is a Caribbean nation whose richly varied local cuisine reflects the country's African, Indian, Spanish, French, Creole, British, Chinese, and Syrian-Lebanese traditions. Living in Maryland, Issa still eats many of the traditional foods he did in his homeland, but some foods, like iguana, goat, rabbit, and wild meats, less frequently.

Influences on dietary patterns

Across the globe, what people eat is influenced by a variety of multi-level factors that intersect to shape a person's food choices and intake. Cultures have different customs around food and eating, and each person has their own preference and eating style. In addition to food preference, other individual factors, such as age, sex, income, knowledge, and cooking skills, can determine food choices. Between the social and cultural influences and the individual factors, a man's diet can also be shaped by his environment (HHS/USDA, 2015). The Social-Ecological Model for Food & Physical Activity Decisions from the Dietary Guidelines for Americans (Figure 13.2) illustrates how there are multiple layers of external and internal forces influencing dietary choices, physical activity patterns, and ultimately health outcomes (HHS/USDA, 2015). The outermost layer of influence in the model is *social and cultural norms and values*. Examples include a person's belief systems, traditions, priorities, lifestyle, and body image. Within the social and cultural context, there are system-wide, organization-level, and industry influences which are referred to as *sectors* in the model. For example, a person's interaction with systems, government, education, health care, or transportation determines his ability to access healthy food. Businesses and industries, notably agriculture, retail, marketing, and media, also influence the food available in communities and what foods and beverages are marketed to the community. Nutrition advocates have raised public awareness about how food companies

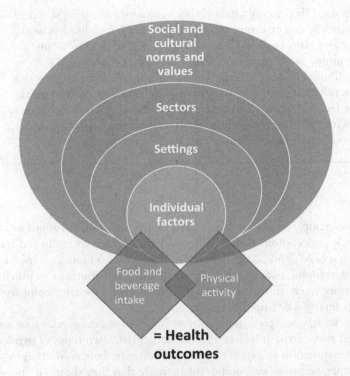

Figure 13.2 A Social-Ecological Model for food and physical activity decisions. The model shows how various factors influence food and beverage intake, physical activity patterns, and ultimately health outcomes.

Source: Adapted from *The Dietary Guidelines for Americans 2015–2020* (HHS/USDA, 2015· Figure 3-1, A Social-Ecological Model for Food and Physical Activity Decisions). Accessed August 2019.

target advertisements for unhealthy foods to low-income communities and communities of color, which contributes to the health disparities across race/ethnicity and socio-economic status (Robert Wood Johnson Foundation, 2019). *Settings* are places where people live, learn, work, play, pray, eat, and conduct other daily activities. The innermost layer of the model is the *individual factors* such as a person's demographics, knowledge, skills, gene–environment interactions, and personal food preferences. Collectively these influences shape a person's day-to-day dietary and physical activity habits, which, over time, influence a person's health outcomes. Public health professionals use the Social-Ecological Model to understand the forces shaping food and activity choices in order to develop effective strategies to positively impact those choices to improve health outcomes.

In his own words

Issa's story

Issa's food and physical activity habits are shaped by many forces that span the Social-Ecological Model. The traditions and cuisine of his mother country (Trinidad and Tobago), food retail environment in his neighborhood in Maryland, food availability at work, his work schedule (currently he works 6:00 a.m.–2:00 p.m.), body image, chronic disease, and unique food preferences all play a role in Issa's day-to-day choices and overall dietary pattern. His personal characteristics influence his meal schedule. "I'm lazy," he says, "so I usually end up eating two big meals a day. It feels like less work." Issa feels like his gender also plays a role in his food choices. "I will not buy a cupcake. To me that is a very feminine food" (personal communication, February 2018).

Since moving to the United States, the biggest change in Issa's eating habits is that he eats out more frequently than he did in Trinidad and Tobago, especially at quick-service restaurants. For Issa, his approach to nutrition is to find a balance between a healthy diet that allows him to manage his chronic condition and support a long life, while also enjoying food as part of social time with friends and family.

Nutrition and gender

Just as every society, ethnic group, and culture has its own beliefs and customs about food, each has its own gender role expectations. Gender roles vary from group to group and can change over time (Oniang'o & Mukudi, 2002). They also interact with biological roles to affect nutrition status. In developing countries, gender inequality contributes to an imbalance in which men are more likely to have good nutrition and food security compared to women and children (Oniang'o & Mukudi, 2002).

Gender stereotypes are widely accepted judgments or biases based on gender that are generally overly simplified and untrue (Planned Parenthood, 2018). Two types of gender stereotypes that can impact nutrition and men's health are domestic behaviors and physical appearance. For example, common stereotypes for men are that they should be muscular, enjoy grilling, and play sports. Gender stereotypes are harmful because they don't allow people to fully express themselves (Planned Parenthood, 2018). They can set men up for unrealistic expectations and result in unequal treatment, both of which can negatively impact food choices and healthy behaviors (see Figure 13.3).

National perspective

In the United States, like many other places around the globe, the greatest nutritional challenges are chronic diseases, including heart disease, cancer, and stroke, and obesity. According to the Centers for Disease Control and Prevention ([CDC], 2019a), in the United States six in every ten adults have a chronic disease, and four in ten have two or more chronic diseases. Chronic disease and obesity rates vary by race/ethnicity and sex. Heart disease is the leading cause of death for men of most racial and ethnic groups in the United States, killing 347,879 men in 2017 (one in every four male deaths) (CDC, 2019b). This suggests that it is especially important for men to follow a dietary pattern that supports heart health.

The United States has the highest rates of overweight and obesity in the world. More than two-thirds of adults and nearly one-third of children and youth are overweight or obese (HHS/USDA, 2015). Rising rates of childhood and adult obesity have led to widespread concerns ranging from the economic costs to national security (CDC, 2019c). For example, the largest reason for disqualification from the military is poor health and fitness (CDC, 2019c). Obesity among active duty military service members in the United States has risen 73% between 2011 and 2015, and 71% of youth can't qualify to join the military (CDC, 2019c). Men in the military are more likely to be overweight and obese than women in the military (Meadows et al., 2018).

How to fight nutrition gender stereotypes

Breaking down gender stereotypes about food and nutrition allows everyone to feel valued and achieve their health goals:

Point it out: Media is full of negative gender stereotypes, but they can sometimes be hard to see unless they are pointed out. Talk with friends and family members about the stereotypes you see and help others understand how sexism and gender stereotypes can be hurtful. While most people recognize that stereotypes are untrue, many still make assumptions based on gender.

Be a living example: Be a role model for your friends and family. Don't let gender stereotypes stop you from eating certain foods or participating in healthy eating behaviors like cooking, eating fruits and vegetables, reading food labels, and paying attention to portion sizes. Encourage others to express themselves and their true qualities through their food and physical activity choices regardless of what society's gender stereotypes and expectations are.

Speak up: If someone is making sexist jokes and comments, whether online or in person, challenge them. For example, someone labeling vegetarian dietary pattern "feminine" implies an imperative to eat meat in order to be masculine. Challenge this assumption and make them aware of these gendered social expectations. Always be respectful and allow for meaningful dialog on all sides.

Give it a try: If you want to do something that's not normally associated with your gender, give it a try. People will learn from your example.

Figure 13.3 How to fight nutrition gender stereotypes.
Source: Adapted from Planned Parenthood (2018). Retrieved from www.plannedparenthood.org/learn/sexual-orientation-gender/gender-gender-identity/what-are-gender-roles-and-stereotypes.

Among adult men in the U.S., the overall prevalence of obesity (BMI greater than 30) is 34% (Ogden et al., 2017). Obesity, like other chronic diseases, disproportionately affects vulnerable groups of people in the United States, including communities of color, communities with high poverty, and adults with lower education levels (Robert Wood Johnson Foundation, 2019). This is an example of a health disparity. Statistics from the CDC (2018) state that Hispanics and non-Hispanic blacks have the highest age-adjusted prevalence of obesity, followed by non-Hispanic whites and non-Hispanic Asians. A recent analysis of the association between obesity and income or educational level found that men with college degrees had lower obesity rates compared to those with less education (Ogden et al., 2017).

Ongoing research continues to explore the root causes of these troubling trends in chronic disease, but changes in dietary patterns and physical activity certainly play a role. Many Americans are eating too many calories and nutrients of concern (including sugar, salt, and fat), in comparison to nutritional needs, and not meeting the recommendations for physical activity (HHS/USDA, 2015). In 2013, 75% of adult men did not meet the guidelines for aerobic and muscle-strengthening recommendations (HHS/USDA, 2015).

Nutritional status of American men

The *2015–2020 Dietary Guidelines for Americans* emphasize that most Americans need to make shifts in their eating patterns to align with healthy eating recommendations. The guidelines recommend consuming a healthy eating pattern that includes a variety of foods from the food groups and subgroups in nutrient-dense forms within an appropriate calorie level. Although American males meet or exceed the recommended intake for protein foods, most fail to meet recommendations for vegetables, fruit, dairy, and whole grains (HHS/USDA, 2015).

Nutritional needs are determined by individual factors including age, sex, and activity level. There are nutrition recommendations for macro and micronutrients, as well as dietary patterns based on food groups. Macronutrients are energy-producing nutrients, which include carbohydrates, protein, and fat. These are required in large amounts in the diet, compared to micronutrients which are chemical elements or substances, such as vitamins and minerals, required in trace amounts for growth and development (USDA, 2019).

The energy and macronutrient nutrition recommendations for men age 19–30 years are included in Table 13.1. Macronutrient recommendations are shown in grams and as a percentage of daily calorie intake. Although each macronutrient provides unique benefits for human health, there are risks when they are over or under consumed compared to the nutritional goals.

Table 13.1 Daily nutritional goals★ for males ages 19–30 years and relevance of macronutrients to men's health

Amounts recommended per day in grams (g) and percent of daily calories (% kcal)	*Nutritional goal*	*Men's health benefits/risks*
Calories (kcal)	2,400–3,000 *Recommendations vary based on activity level.*	**Benefits:** Calories are the energy people get from the food and beverages they consume. The human body converts the potential energy of nutrients to usable chemical energy (HHS/USDA, 2015). **Risks:** Calorie balance (calories consumed compared to calories expended) impacts weight. A calorie imbalance where more calories are consumed than expended can lead to weight gain over time, and is contributing to the high prevalence of overweight and obesity.
Macronutrients Carbohydrate, g (% kcal)	130 (45–65%)	**Benefits:** Carbohydrates are the main source of energy in the diet. They provide the body with glucose, which is converted to usable energy. Healthy sources of carbohydrates include whole grains, vegetables, fruits, and beans (USDA, 2019). **Risks:** Unhealthy sources of carbohydrates common in the American diet include white bread, pastries, sugar-sweetened beverages or other highly processed foods. When consumed in higher than recommended amounts, these foods can replace nutrient-dense foods in the diet and may contribute to weight gain, promote diabetes and heart disease (HHS/USDA, 2015).
Added sugars, % kcal	<10%	**Risks:** Added sugars are one of the nutrients of concern in the *Dietary Guidelines* because of how many excess calories they contribute to the typical American diet. Intakes are especially high among children, adolescents, and young adults. Added sugars account for 17% of calories per day for teen boys, compared to the *Dietary Guidelines* maximum limit of 10% of calories (HHS/USDA, 2015). The largest source of added sugars in the American diet is sugary drinks, which include soft drinks, fruit drinks, sweetened coffee and tea, energy drinks, alcoholic beverages, and flavored water (HHS/USDA, 2015). Consumption of sugary drinks can lead to obesity, diabetes, tooth decay, and heart disease (Center for Science in the Public Interest, 2018).

Table 13.1 Cont.

Amounts recommended per day in grams (g) and percent of daily calories (% kcal)	Nutritional goal	Men's health benefits/risks
Protein, g (% kcal)	56 (10–35%)	**Benefits:** Protein (amino acids) is the building block of much of the human body. The body uses protein to build and repair tissues, make enzymes, hormones, and other body chemicals (USDA, 2019). **Risks:** American men meet or exceed the recommendations for protein intake. Many foods rich in protein (such as beef, nuts, and cheese) are also high in fat. Thus a high-protein diet may exceed the recommended limits for fat intake if the majority of protein sources are not lean protein foods (such as poultry, tuna fish, low-fat dairy, or eggs). High-protein/low-carbohydrate diets can change metabolism and experts caution that these changes may have long-term health consequences (Harvard T.H. Chan School of Public Health, 2019).
Total fat, % kcal Saturated fat, %kcal	20–35% <10%	**Benefits:** Fat is a necessary nutrient in the human diet to provide energy, support growth, produce hormones, and help the body absorb some nutrients. Unsaturated fats (liquid fats like oil) can lower bad cholesterol levels and are beneficial for brain health (USDA, 2019). **Risks:** American men exceed the recommendations for fat and saturated fat intake among all age groups. Fat has more than twice as many calories per gram as carbohydrates and protein, so overconsumption of total fat can result in excess calorie intake and weight gain (USDA, 2019). Saturated fat and *trans fats* (solid fats at room temperature, such as butter) raise bad cholesterol levels in the blood and increase the risk for cardiovascular disease (USDA, 2019).

Notes:
★ Nutritional goals based on dietary reference intakes and *Dietary Guidelines* recommendations (HHS/USDA, 2015).
For a full list of nutritional goals by age-sex groups, including vitamins and minerals, visit: https://health.gov/dietaryguidelines/2015/guidelines/appendix-7/.
Source: Developed by chapter author.

Food and nutrient labeling

Nutrition labels are used globally as an informational tool that can encourage healthy eating habits. In the United States, the nutrition label is called the Nutrition Facts panel. The Nutrition Facts panel has been required on most packaged foods in the United States since the passage of the Nutritional Labeling and Education Act of 1990 (Food and Drug Administration [FDA], 2017). In May 2016, the FDA released rules to update the Nutrition Facts panel format and content (FDA, 2017). The updated Nutrition Facts highlights added sugars, enlarges total calories, and makes serving sizes more reflective of serving sizes usually consumed (Figure 13.4). Research has consistently

Nutrition Facts

Serving Size 2/3 cup (55g)

Servings Per Container About 8

Amount Per Serving

Calories 230   Calories from Fat 72

                                              % Daily Value*

Total Fat 8g	12%
Saturated Fat 1g	5%
Trans Fat 0g	
Cholesterol 0mg	0%
Sodium 160mg	7%
Total Carbohydrate 37g	12%
Dietary Fiber 4g	16%
Sugars 1g	
Protein 3g	

Vitamin A	10%
Vitamin C	8%
Calcium	20%
Iron	45%

*Percent Daily Values are based on a 2,000 calorie diet. Your daily value may be higher or lower depending on your calorie needs.

	Calories:	2,000	2,500
Total Fat	Less than	65g	80g
Sat Fat	Less than	20g	25g
Cholesterol	Less than	300mg	300mg
Sodium	Less than	2,400mg	2,400mg
Total Carbohydrate		300g	375g
Dietary Fiber		25g	30g

Nutrition Facts

8 servings per container

Serving Size   2/3 cup (55g)

Amount Per Serving

Calories   **230**

                                              % Daily Value*

Total Fat 8g	10%
Saturated Fat 1g	5%
Trans Fat 0g	
Cholesterol 0mg	0%
Sodium 160mg	7%
Total Carbohydrate 37g	13%
Dietary Fiber 4g	14%
Total Sugars 12g	
Includes 10g Added Sugars	**20%**
Protein 3g	

Vitamin D 2mcg	10%
Calcium 260mg	20%
Iron 8mg	45%
Potassium 235mg	6%

*The % Daily Value (DV) tells you how much a nutrient in a serving of food contributes to a daily diet. 2,000 calories a day is used for general nutrition advice.

Figure 13.4 Side-by-side comparison of the original and new formats of the Nutrition Facts panel. *Source*: Food and Drug Administration (2017).

shown the use of the Nutrition Facts panel on packaged foods is lower among men than women (Cowburn & Stockley, 2005). Results from the Project EAT-IV (Eating and Activity in Teens and Young Adults) study showed that only 26% of male study participants reported using the Nutrition Facts panel "most of the time" and "always" when buying or choosing a food product for the first time, and women were significantly more likely than men to look at information on sugars, fibers, and calories from fat (Christoph, Larson, Laska, & Neumark-Sztainer, 2018). Since men exhibit lower label use than women, men should be particularly supported and educated on nutrient label use and interpretation. Health professionals can encourage the use of Nutrition Facts when choosing products and support men in appropriately understanding this information. Men can leverage the Nutrition Facts panel as a way to help ensure proper nutrient intake for their physical activity level, which could potentially promote healthier dietary patterns.

Nutrition mobile apps

With the rise in the popularity of mobile devices, there has been an increase in the availability and popularity of nutrition software applications for mobile devices (i.e. apps) to support healthy eating and weight management. There are many benefits to using apps: they are generally low or no cost, accessible anytime, and can provide different types of support to users (e.g., behavior self-monitoring or social support). Nutrition mobile apps can be used to count calories, inform healthy choices at point of purchase at restaurants or grocery stores, better understand nutrition labels, or find products that meet dietary restrictions. For example, the Fooducate Diet & Nutrition app (free on iOS and Android) lets you scan nutrition labels for a quick assessment of how healthy something is and can recommend healthier alternatives. Nutrition apps can provide an easier way to record dietary intake and exercise than pen and paper. Many have goal-setting features based on calorie and nutrient recommendations that can increase the success of achieving nutritional or weight loss goals. An example is the MyFitnessPal mobile app which allows users to set a daily calorie goal and record daily food and exercise to help them stay on track with their goal. This app is available in several countries, and can be tailored to local language and foods (Ha, 2014). However, the effectiveness of using apps for weight loss, weight maintenance, or weight gain compared to other methods is still emerging. The adherence to self-monitoring using apps can be challenging, and requires self-motivation for effective app use. For recommendations and reviews of nutrition apps, visit foodandnutrition. org/tag/apps.

Nutrition mobile apps are a low-cost, convenient tool to use to assess eating habits and knowledge. Apps can help users track calories, nutrients, or food groups. By comparing eating patterns to health recommendations, users can assess whether they are meeting the healthy eating recommendations and identify areas to make a change. Many apps allow users to set goals, such as a target weight, and provide feedback on whether you are making progress toward achieving the goal based on current habits. Individuals seeking professional assistance with nutrition assessment and making dietary changes can work with a Registered Dietitian (RD) or Registered Dietitian Nutritionist (RDN). ChooseMyPlate. gov also provides tools for dietary assessment, nutrition education, and nutrition quizzes for users to test their nutrition knowledge.

Nutrition health professionals

The health care system plays an important role in improving men's nutrition. Primary care providers are responsible for completing recommended preventive health screenings and treatment. For example, the U.S. Preventive Services Task Force (USPSTF) recommends screening all adults for obesity, and that clinicians should offer or refer patients who are overweight or obese, and have additional cardiovascular disease risk factors, to intensive behavioral counseling interventions to promote a healthful diet and physical activity (USPFTF, 2018). Intensive behavioral therapy can include programs with different modes of delivery (e.g., phone, internet, or face-to-face). The Affordable Care Act requires health insurance plans to cover nutritional counseling at no cost (for in-network providers) for people who are overweight or have specific health risks, based on a recommendation by the USPSTF (2018).

Food and nutrition experts, RDs or RDNs, can provide preventive and medical nutrition therapy services in a variety of settings, including health care facilities, home health care, food service, business, research, and educational organizations. They can help individuals make personalized, positive lifestyle changes to improve health or fight disease. RDs and RDNs can also help with creating personalized meal plans that meet a person's dietary needs, dietary restrictions, and personal food and beverage preferences. RDs and RDNs are trusted sources for food and nutrition information and can provide guidance on topics ranging from sports nutrition and supplements to food–medication interactions or diet trends. On college campuses, nutritional counseling is commonly available as part of college health services. To find an RD or RDN in your area, visit www.eatright.org/find-an-expert.

Nutrition education and meal planning

The 2015–2020 edition of the *Dietary Guidelines* emphasizes healthy eating patterns, rather than specific food groups or nutrients, because it is the totality of the diet that most strongly correlates to health outcomes over time, rather than individual nutrients. The *Dietary Guidelines* define a healthy U.S.-Style Eating Pattern as one that exemplifies healthy eating based on the types and proportions of foods Americans typically consume, but in nutrient-dense forms and appropriate amounts, designed to meet nutrient needs while not exceeding calorie requirements (HHS/USDA, 2015).

The *Dietary Guidelines* is the basis for the federal public nutrition education materials, based on MyPlate (Figure 13.5), that inform nutrition education in schools, health care, and nutrition programs across the country (HHS/USDA, 2015). MyPlate is a symbol that serves as a reminder to build healthy eating patterns by making healthy choices across the five food groups: fruits, vegetables, grains, protein, and dairy. The website Choosemyplate. gov offers resources to help consumers determine what and how much to eat.

One of the nutrition education tools available in English and Spanish on Choosemyplate.gov is the MyPlate Plan. This shows your food group targets – what and how much to eat within your calorie allowance. Your food plan is personalized, based on your age, sex, height, weight, and physical activity level. The plan includes the estimated calorie needs per day, and daily recommended amounts for each food group.

The sample meal plan in this chapter shows an example of the healthy U.S.-Style Eating Pattern in the *Dietary Guidelines* and how the MyPlate Plan shown can be translated into snacks and meals. The sample meal plans provide options that can be customized to accommodate cultural, ethnic, traditional, and personal preference. To create your MyPlate Plan, visit www.choosemyplate.gov/MyPlatePlan. For additional meal planning information, visit www.cdc.gov/healthyweight/healthy_eating/meals.html.

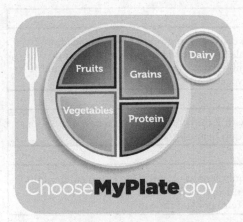

Figure 13.5 Choosemyplate.gov. The MyPlate icon replaced the food pyramid as the symbol of the USDA's food guidance for Americans since 2011. It was introduced along with updating of USDA food patterns for the 2010 Dietary Guidelines for Americans. The icon serves as a reminder for healthy eating.

Source: U.S. Department of Agriculture.

In his own words

Issa's story

Like many people, Issa aspires to eat healthfully. "I want to live a long life for my family. I'm a father now and I want to be around a long time for my daughter. With Crohn's Disease, I also have to pay attention to what I eat because it makes me feel more comfortable and allows me to function day-to-day" (personal communication, February 2018). Issa's main barrier to achieving his nutrition and physical activity goals is time. He is working full-time and taking classes on Saturdays. In his words, "I'm so busy right now and I would rather be with my daughter than go to the gym, especially after work" (personal communication, February 2018). Another barrier is frequent gatherings with family and friends often include unhealthy foods. Issa does his best to balance his enjoyment of food and drink at these gatherings with concerns about the effect on his gut or long-term health.

Sample meal plan for Issa
This 2,400 calorie meal plan provides options for a healthy dietary pattern specifically recommended for people with diet restrictions due to ulcerative colitis or Crohn's Disease.
Breakfast:
■ 2 eggs or ½ cup egg substitute (= 2 ounces of protein) scrambled with 1.5 ounces low-fat cheddar cheese (= 1 cup of dairy)
■ 2 slices potato bread (= 2 ounces equivalent of grains)
■ 1 cup watermelon (= 1 cup of fruit)
Snack:
■ 1 cup (8 ounces) plain Greek yogurt (= 1 cup of dairy) with ½ cup diced cantaloupe (= ½ cup fruit)

Lunch:
■ 4 ounces (= 4 ounces equivalent protein) cooked lean ground turkey divided on 2 (8-inch) flour tortillas (= 2 ounces equivalent of grains) topped with 1 medium avocado (= 3 teaspoons of oil), 2 pieces Bibb lettuce (= ½ cup of vegetables) and ½ cup mild salsa (as tolerated) (= ½ cup of vegetables)
Snack:
■ 1 large banana (= 1 cup of fruit) spread with 2 tbsp creamy nut butter (= 4 teaspoons of oil) and 1 ounce pretzels (= 1 ounce equivalent of grains)
Dinner:
■ 1 cup cooked penne pasta (= 2 ounces equivalent of grains) with 1 tbsp extra virgin olive oil (= 3 teaspoons of oil), fresh herbs, 1 cup well-cooked spinach (= 1 cup of vegetables) and 3 ounces (= 3 ounces protein) cooked shrimp
■ 1 cup unsweetened calcium fortified soy milk (= 1 cup dairy). Cow's milk or other milk can be used.
Nutrition Facts:
Calories: 2,411 Total Fat: 102 grams Saturated Fat: 13 grams Protein: 127 grams Carbohydrates: 256 grams Total Sugars: 64 grams Fiber: 26 grams

Figure 13.6 Sample meal plan for Issa.

Source: Menu adapted from www.crohnscolitisfoundation.org/sites/default/files/legacy/assets/pdfs/diet-nutrition-2013.pdf.

Nutrition Facts information from: Myfitnesspal.com.

Developed by chapter author.

Supplements

The *Dietary Guidelines* recommend that individuals meet nutritional needs primarily through foods (HHS/USDA, 2015). Foods in nutrient-dense forms contain essential vitamins, minerals, dietary fiber, and other naturally occurring substances (such as antioxidants) that have positive health effects. In some cases, fortified foods and dietary supplements may be useful in providing one or more nutrients that otherwise may be consumed in less than recommended amounts. For example, healthcare providers may prescribe an iron supplement for someone with an iron deficiency.

Dietary supplements are defined and regulated by the FDA under the Dietary Supplement Health and Education Act of 1994 (FDA, 2019). The law defines dietary supplements in part as products taken by mouth that contain a dietary ingredient, including vitamins, minerals, amino acids, herbs, or enzymes (FDA, 2019). They can be marketed in forms such as tablets, capsules, softgels, gelcaps, powders, and liquids. Some common dietary supplements include fish oil, glucosamine, echinacea, calcium, and ginseng. To protect the public from misleading marketing, the FDA prohibits supplements from being marketed for treating or preventing disease (FDA, 2019). So supplements cannot make health claims, such as "lowers high cholesterol" or "treats heart disease." However, the FDA is not authorized to review dietary supplements for safety and effectiveness before they are marketed (FDA, 2019). This means that the risks in taking supplements are two-fold: (1) the active ingredients in supplements could have a biological effect that could hurt or complicate health under certain conditions, especially if taken in large quantities; and (2) supplements could contain contaminants, impurities, or be found to be unsafe since they are not reviewed for safety or effectiveness before they are marketed. Some dietary supplements have sufficient evidence to show therapeutic benefit, but many do not. Despite the common practice of taking large doses of vitamin C to prevent a cold, evidence shows that vitamin C supplementation does not reduce the occurrence of colds in the general population (Cochrane Complementary Medicine, 2019). However, research does suggest that taking vitamin C supplementation or echinacea (*Echinacea purpurea*) after the onset of a cold can help reduce the duration and severity of the cold (Cochrane Complementary Medicine, 2019).

Consumers should research supplements on noncommercial sites (e.g. NIH, FDA, USDA), and be wary of supplement claims. Consumers should talk to their healthcare provider about supplements they are considering to determine if they would be safe and beneficial.

Conclusion

Improving nutrition requires a collection of strategies, implemented across the levels of the Social-Ecological Model, to create environments that promote health and shift people's eating habits for the better. As an example, ChangeLab Solutions (2018) developed a Sugar-Sweetened Beverages Playbook which provides ten strategies to reduce sugary beverage consumption through policies, sectors, settings, communities, and individual action (Figure 13.7).

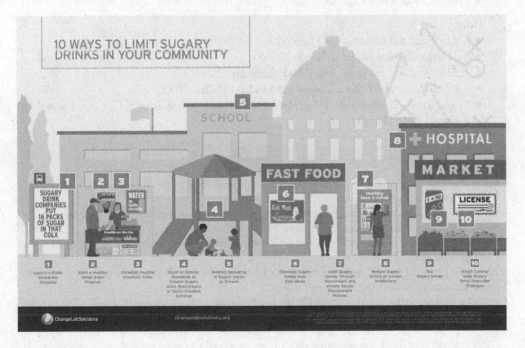

Figure 13.7 Ten ways to limit sugary drinks in your community. Strategies to reduce sugary beverage consumption.

Source: Illustrations by Black Graphics, courtesy of ChangeLab Solutions, used with permission.

Individuals have many potential options to improve their own nutritional status, such as using the Nutrition Facts panel to make healthier food choices or using a mobile app to assess their calorie input and expenditure. However, substantial and sustained improvements in men's health requires changes at all levels of the Social-Ecological Model. Institutions can implement healthy vending options to make healthy food options more widely available at businesses and worksites. Hospitals and health leaders in the community can promote and expand access to nutrition education and counseling, and healthcare facilities can remove unhealthy food from facility concessions and vending. Cities and states can leverage policy options to limit unhealthy food marketing, set pricing strategies such as raising taxes on unhealthy food items, adopting nutrition standards for public places such as government buildings and parks, and creating media messages to promote consumer awareness of good nutrition (Public Health Law Center, 2019). Good nutrition is a key strategy for national and global leaders to support people to attain the highest level of health possible.

Book and movie recommendations

The following is a list of recommended movie documentaries and books to learn more:

Documentaries
- *Supersize Me*
- *Fat, Sick and Nearly Dead*
- *Food Inc.*
- *Forks Over Knives*

Books
- *On Food and Cooking* by Harold McGee (2004)
- *What to Eat* by Marion Nestle (2008)
- *How to Cook Everything* by Mark Bittman (2008)
- *Food Rules: An Eater's Manual* by Michael Pollan (2009)
- *The Truth About Food: Why Pandas Eat Bamboo and People Get Bamboozled* by David Katz (2018)

References

Centers for Disease Control and Prevention. (2018). *Adult obesity facts.* Retrieved from www.cdc.gov/obesity/data/adult.html

Centers for Disease Control and Prevention. (2019a). *About chronic disease.* Retrieved from www.cdc.gov/chronicdisease/about/index.htm

Centers for Disease Control and Prevention. (2019b). *Men and heart disease.* Retrieved from www.cdc.gov/heartdisease/men.htm

Centers for Disease Control and Prevention. (2019c). *Unfit to serve.* Retrieved from www.cdc.gov/physicalactivity/downloads/unfit-to-serve.pdf

Center for Science in the Public Interest. (2018). *Local sugary drink taxes voted on 2014–2017.* Retrieved from https://cspinet.org/resource/local-sugary-drink-taxes-voted-2014%E2%80%932017

ChangeLab Solutions. (2018). *10 ways to limit sugary drinks in your community. Updated September 2018.* Retrieved from www.changelabsolutions.org/product/sugary-drink-strategy-playbook

Cochrane Complementary Medicine. (2019). *Common cold.* Retrieved from https://cam.cochrane.org/common-cold

Christoph, M. J., Larson, N., Laska, M. N., & Neumark-Sztainer, D. (2018). Nutrition facts panels: Who uses them, what do they use, and how does use relate to dietary intake? *Journal of the Academy of Nutrition and Dietetics, 118*(2), 217–228. doi: 10.1016/j.jand.2017.10.014

Cowburn, G., & Stockley, L. (2005). Consumer understanding and use of nutrition labelling: A systematic review. *Public Health Nutrition, 8*(1), 21–28. doi: 10.1079/PHN2004666.

Development Initiatives (2018). *2018 Global Nutrition Report: Shining a light to spur action on nutrition.* Bristol, UK: Development Initiatives. Retrieved from https://globalnutritionreport.org/

Food and Drug Administration. (2017). *Changes to the nutrition facts label.* Retrieved from www.fda.gov/food/food-labeling-nutrition/changes-nutrition-facts-label

Food and Drug Administration. (2019). *Information for consumers on using dietary supplements.* Retrieved from www.fda.gov/food/dietary-supplements/information-consumers-using-dietary-supplements

Ha, A. (2014). *MyFitnessPal moves into Asia with localized apps for China, Japan, and Korea.* Retrieved from https://techcrunch.com/2014/05/02/myfitnesspal-asian-expansion/

Harvard T.H. Chan School of Public Health. (2019). The nutrition source: Low-carbohydrate diets. Retrieved from www.hsph.harvard.edu/nutritionsource/carbohydrates/low-carbohydrate-diets/

Meadows, S. O., Engel, C. C., Collins, R. L., Beckman, R. L., Cefalu, M., Hawes-Dawson, J., … Williams, K. M. (2018). *2015 Department of Defense Health Related Behaviors Survey (HRBS),* Santa Monica, CA: RAND Corporation, RR-1695-OSD, 2018. Retrieved from www.rand.org/pubs/research_reports/RR1695.html

Ogden, C. L., Fakhouri, T. H., Carroll, M. D., Hales, C. M., Fryar, C. D., Li, X., & Freeman, D. S. (2017). Prevalence of obesity among adults, by household income and education — United States, 2011–2014. *Morbidity and Mortality Weekly Report, 6,* 1369–1373. doi: http://dx.doi.org/10.15585/mmwr.mm6650a1

Oniang'o, R., & Mukudi, E. (2002). Nutrition and gender. In *Nutrition: A Foundation for Development,* Geneva: ACC/SCN. Retrieved from www.unscn.org/files/Publications/Briefs_on_Nutrition/Brief7_EN.pdf.

Planned Parenthood. (2018). *What are gender roles and stereotypes?* Retrieved from www.plannedparenthood.org/learn/sexual-orientation-gender/gender-gender-identity/what-are-gender-roles-and-stereotypes

Public Health Law Center. (2019). *Healthy eating.* Retrieved from www.publichealthlawcenter.org/topics/healthy-eating

Robert Wood Johnson Foundation. (2019). *State of obesity.* Retrieved from www.stateofobesity.org/

U.S. Department of Agriculture. (2019). *Food and nutrition information center.* Retrieved from www.nal.usda.gov/fnic/macronutrients

U.S. Department of Health and Human Services and U.S. Department of Agriculture. (2015). *2015–2020 Dietary Guidelines for Americans.* 8th Edition. Retrieved from https://health.gov/dietaryguidelines/2015/guidelines/

U.S. Department of Health and Human Services. (2018). *Physical Activity Guidelines for Americans, 2nd edition.* Washington, DC: U.S. Department of Health and Human Services. Retrieved from https://health.gov/paguidelines/second-edition/

U.S. Preventive Services Task Force. (September 2018). *Final update summary: Weight loss to prevent obesity-related morbidity and mortality in adults: Behavioral interventions.* Retrieved from www.uspreventiveservicestaskforce.org/Page/Document/UpdateSummaryFinal/obesity-in-adults-interventions1

World Health Organization. (2019a). *Noncommunicable diseases (NCD).* Retrieved from www.who.int/gho/ncd/en/

World Health Organization. (2019b). *Nutrition.* Retrieved from www.who.int/topics/nutrition/en/

14 Physical fitness/activity

Kayla K. McDonald

Physical activity, or any movement of the body that burns calories, is an important part of living a healthy lifestyle (Mayo Clinic, 2005). Physical activity includes regular daily or weekly activities, such as mowing the lawn, walking the dog, gardening, and even taking the stairs. Physical activity extends to exercise, but exercise is not the exclusive form of physical activity (Mayo Clinic, 2005). The movement of the body plays a role in increasing longevity and decreasing the risk of numerous chronic diseases. Throughout life, physical activity varies based on the individual and many influencing factors, including: the phase of their life, the environment that they live in, their mobility, their interests, and underlying conditions, among other factors.

Recommended levels of physical activity

The Centers for Disease Control and Prevention (CDC) recommends that all individuals participate in 150 minutes of physical activity each week (Centers for Disease Control and Prevention [CDC], 2019). While these guidelines are recommended by the CDC (2017), in addition to the World Health Organization (WHO, 2018a), it is reported that only about half (53.3%) of adults in the U.S. meet the expectation. The WHO (2018a) reports that globally one in four adults are not active enough to see the benefits of physical activity. More specifically, across the globe, men are more active than women (Guthold, Stevens, Riley, & Bull, 2018). In fact, across all regions in the world, except for east and southeast Asia, men are more physically active than women (Guthold et al., 2018).

The consensus provided among the WHO (2018a) is that the recommended 150 minutes of physical activity each week should be of moderate intensity. If the individual participates in vigorous or intense physical activity, then 75 minutes each week would suffice (WHO, 2018a). It is important to note that this is the recommended minimum number of minutes, for additional health benefits and reducing the risk of a variety of chronic conditions, adults should increase their moderate-intensity physical activity to 300 minutes per week (WHO, 2018a). Moderate activities include activities where you can talk while doing them, such as gardening, ballroom dancing, walking briskly, and doubles tennis. Vigorous activities include those that you can only say a few words without stopping to catch your breath, such as running, singles tennis, Zumba, and hiking uphill (Hales, 2017).

Physical activity should be diverse in the muscle groups being worked on and the type of activity. Various muscle groups often relate to the region of the body that is being worked. The seven major muscle groups include: chest, legs and calves, shoulders, back, front of arms, back of arms, and abdominals (commonly referred to as abs). It is encouraged by the WHO (2018a) that muscle-strengthening should take place at least two days per week. Macmillan Support Group (2016), a support system based out of England that focuses on living a healthier life, provides a realistic approach to completing 150 minutes of physical activity each week. As seen in Figure 14.1, the activities selected include everyday activities and exercises, but also include various movements that would work different muscle groups within the body (Macmillan Support Group, 2016). By diversifying the activities completed, the greater the likelihood of seeing a positive outcome from physical activity throughout the entire body.

Though diversifying activities is recommended, there are activities that are stereotyped as being less masculine. An example of this would be yoga. There are great benefits to yoga, such as improving flexibility, balance, breathing, and mental space, but the current global culture of yoga consists of approximately 80 percent women (Remski, 2017). Looking back at the origins of yoga, it was primarily practiced by men and was not particularly welcoming to women (Remski, 2017). This shift in the stereotype occurred in the mid-1900s, though there has been a recent shift back in the acceptance of men in yoga and the acceptance of yoga by men (Tilin, 2017). The stereotype is being addressed head on by professional athletes like LeBron James and Tim Thomas to show that the benefits of the practice can present great outcomes for the body and mind (Tilin, 2017).

The value of physical activity

Of course, physical activity helps individuals look and feel good, but it is also a key part to living a healthy life. Living a more active life is related to lowering the risk of heart disease, stroke, type 2 diabetes, high blood pressure, dementia and Alzheimer's, in addition to various kinds of cancer, including prostate cancer (American Heart Association, 2018). Not only can physical activity help to lower the risk of many chronic conditions, it can also help improve sleep, improve cognition, regulate weight fluctuations, build strong muscular and skeletal systems to help improve balance and flexibility, reduce symptoms of depression and anxiety, and improve the quality of life for individuals (American Heart Association, 2018). Physical activity has been linked to helping to boost mood, elevating self-esteem, increasing energy, reducing tension, relieving stress, and improving concentration and alertness (Hales, 2017). Living a physically fit life has been proven to help men live longer, healthier lives and to increase testosterone levels and reduce erectile dysfunction (Mayo Clinic, 2019).

When it comes to physical activity, the quality of the way the body moves, is just as important as the amount of time that is spent being active. The way the body is exerted through various activities plays a vital role in reducing the risk factors associated with chronic illnesses (Mayo Clinic, 2005). With quality and quantity as significant factors to remember in physical activity, recognizing that both play a role in the outcome of one's health is vital. Obtaining optimal health is multifaceted and physical activity is one key part of reaching toward living a healthy life.

Consistency in physical activity is also an important factor in attainment of the maximum benefits of exercise. While 150 to 300 minutes of diversified physical activity are recommended per week, this effort should be spread throughout the week and should be consistent from week to week. Completing 150 minutes of physical activity on Monday

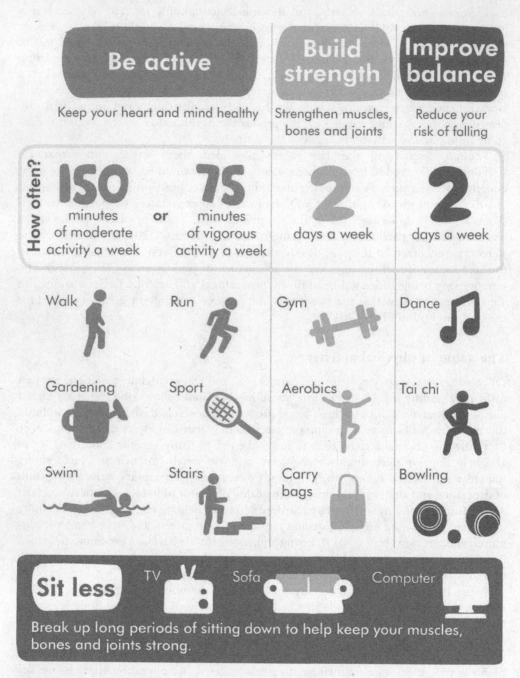

Figure 14.1 Completing 150 minutes of physical activity each week.

Source: This image was produced by Macmillan Cancer Support and is reused with permission.

followed by very little movement the remainder of the week will have limited health benefits. It is the same concept as working out one day then waiting three weeks before working out again and expecting our bodies to get stronger. We must put the effort in each day to see the short- and long-term benefits.

Implementing and maintaining a life full of physical activity

Ideas that often stand in between individuals and being physically active typically include lack of time, not being interested in physical activity, lacking motivation, physical ability, and the weather. It can be intimidating to begin a regular routine to increase physical activity and improve the health and well-being of an individual, but scheduling weekly physical activities can help to ensure that you are physically active. It is important to note that individuals cannot be rushed into this behavior change, since this is not an effective strategy toward getting them to participate in a healthier lifestyle (Prochaska & Velicer, 1997). Having the individual set goals can often motivate them to get started and maintain an active lifestyle. Additionally, social support can also play a role in the motivation of an individual to participate in physical activities.

When first beginning to implement intentional physical activity in one's life, it is encouraged to begin small and to remember that this lifelong journey is unique to everyone. Physical activity does not have to include going to the gym, but could include walking or biking to local errands, or parking at the far end of the parking lot at the grocery store to increase the walk. Physical activity extends to walking around the zoo with the children, mowing the yard, and taking a dog on a walk. Beginning with small tasks makes the idea of 150 minutes (two and a half hours) per week seem less daunting. The key to physical activity is getting up and moving, rather than being sedentary. As little as 20 minutes each day, adds up to 140 minutes a week – so even in busy lives, people can find about 20 minutes each day.

The American Council on Exercise recommends good shoes, fun music, free weights, a positive attitude, comfy clothing, adequate water, proper safety/support equipment, well-made equipment, and a workout partner as some of the exercise essentials (Mayo Clinic, 2005). Motivation from peers can encourage individuals to begin living a more active life, and an accountability partner is often encouraged to continue through the lifelong journey of physical activity. Accountability partners may be lifelong, or interchanging based on the activities you are participating in. An example may include meeting a neighbor for a walk every Saturday or attending yoga with your spouse on Wednesdays. Having someone to hold you accountable to your goals is important in working toward being more physically active.

Some forms of physical activity or exercise do require equipment. Common equipment includes free weights, resistance machines, resistance bands, and other gym machines such as treadmills, stationary bicycles, stair masters, and ellipticals (Mayo Clinic, 2005). Safety and proper use of equipment is just as important as having the equipment available for use. To further understand the proper use of a piece of equipment, please be sure to review the manual or to ask a fitness professional for assistance.

Ensuring proper workout gear is important to ensure optimal and comfortable performance. Clothes should be comfortable to wear and move in. Footwear is often specific to the activity that is being done (Mayo Clinic, 2005). It is encouraged that the individual be fitted for the shoe they intend to wear for physical activity. Sizing of a shoe is typically available by a staff member in a shoe department at a retailer or sporting goods store.

To see the greatest effects of physical activity it is important to fuel the body properly. Fueling the body includes adequate nutrition, that is balanced among all food groups (protein, carbohydrates, fats, fruits, vegetables, and dairy). Individuals will also want to ensure adequate hydration. Fueling our bodies prior to and after physical activity is key to reaching the maximum results of physical activity (Mayo Clinic, 2005).

Types of physical activity

There are a variety of ways to engage in physical activity, but the main two types of physical activity are aerobic and anaerobic activities, both of which present unique health benefits. Aerobic activities are known as activities that increase breathing and heart rate for a period of time (Chertoff, 2018). Examples of aerobic exercise include dancing, running, biking, and swimming laps. Aerobic exercise is recommended to take place in three parts:

1. *Warm-up*: which includes stretching, allows the body to adjust to movement and slowly ramp up the heart rate
2. *Conditioning*: the actual movement that you are participating in (usually for 10–60 minutes), generally involves an increase in heart rate compared to the resting heart rate of the individual
3. *Cool-down*: bringing the body back to a normal heart rate and stretching the muscles that have been strained throughout your activity

Aerobic exercise can help to lower and maintain a healthy blood pressure, increase stamina, reduce fatigue, strengthen the heart, and boost mood (Chertoff, 2018).

Anaerobic activities increase the heart rate in quick bursts and can include resistance training, core stability, flexibility, and balance (Mayo Clinic, 2005). These activities are usually done at maximum effort and for a short length of time, like with high intensity interval training (HIIT), jumping, sprinting, or weightlifting (Chertoff, 2018). Benefits of anaerobic exercise include building muscle mass, strengthening bones, burning fat, and increasing stamina for daily activities (Chertoff, 2018).

The combination of aerobic and anaerobic activities in an individual's weekly physical activity is recommended to reach the highest potential of cardiorespiratory fitness (UCHealth, 2016). Individuals don't need to be an athlete to be physically active, but there are individuals who find more pleasure in participating in an organized sport to stay physically active, while others prefer to approach physical activity through their daily activities. There is no right or wrong way to staying physically fit, so long as you are safe and consistent. The location of where you are physically active may vary based on the activity or preference. A common misconception is that you can only be active at the gym, but you can certainly bike around your community, play at a sports field, run around your back yard with your children, or in your home. Physical activity can take place anywhere at any time.

Often, gyms or local recreation centers will provide fitness classes, such as cycling, water aerobics, and yoga. Classes are generally offered at varying levels, from beginners to more proficient or experienced. When considering a fitness facility, it is important to review the location, hours, environment, equipment available, classes, the employees, cost, amenities, any accommodations for special needs, and the affiliation with other centers

(Mayo Clinic, 2005). In addition to recreation centers, many communities work to maintain green space/parks to encourage physical activity. These often include nature trails, bike paths, fields, and sometimes, if near water, even boating, like kayak and canoe, rentals.

Environmental factors play a large role in whether individuals participate in physical activity. Individuals may become discouraged from participating in physical activity if they are exposed to fear of violence or crime, high-density traffic, pollution, or lack of green space (parks, sidewalks, and sports/recreation fields) (WHO, 2018a). To reduce these environmental barriers the WHO (2018a) recommends that countries establish and enforce policies aimed to increase physical activity. Creating safe environments that encourage physically fit lifestyles often reflect in a healthier community, with lower rates of obesity and other related chronic illnesses, such as cardiovascular diseases and type 2 diabetes (WHO, 2018a).

Safety and injury

To prevent injuries from occurring, it is recommended that you avoid overuse of any one muscle group, stretch, leave recovery time between workouts, wear proper equipment, and fuel your body adequately. Warming up and cooling down are key steps in injury prevention. Tips for warming up and cooling down have been included below:

- Before you begin activity begin with walking in place to get your heart rate up
- Begin stretching various parts of your body, never extending any part past their normal range of motion
- Do not hold your breath while stretching, the body still needs oxygen
- Don't make any sudden movements, stretching should feel fluid and comfortable
- Listen to your body, only do what feels comfortable to you

If you have been sedentary for an extended period or live with a chronic condition, it is recommended that you discuss introducing physical activity in your daily life with your physician. Additionally, the idea of *no pain, no gain* is dangerous. Physical activity and exercise should feel good, and no pain should be present. Should an individual feel pain, they should contact their physician. According to the Mayo Clinic (2005), warning signs that should lead an individual to stop immediately, and seek medical attention include:

- Chest pain or tightness
- Dizziness/faintness
- Pain in the arm or jaw
- Severe shortness of breath
- Bursts of very rapid or slow heart rate
- Irregular heartbeat
- Excessive fatigue
- Severe joint or muscle pain
- Joint swelling

With all physical activity there is the possibility of injury. Because of the anatomy of males versus females, there are injuries that are more prevalent in men than women. Some of these include: plantar fasciitis, ankle sprains, knee ligament strain, quad strain, and hamstring pull (Pacific Prime, 2013). As the individual begins to explore the realm of physical activity it is important to remember that the journey is specific to the individual themselves. Beginning simple or small and working up is a safe practice to follow. A good rule when it comes to injuries is that when you feel pain, it is best to follow the acronym RICE:

- R – Rest
- I – Ice
- C – Compress
- E – Elevate

If the swelling and pain do not subside after a few days it is best to contact your primary care physician to have them further evaluate the injury. In some cases, the primary care physician will refer you to a specialist and/or physical therapist to assist in providing the best care for you as the patient. Please note that in case of an emergency, 9-1-1 or your local emergency line should be contacted first.

Engaging in safe practices is just as important as participating in physical activity. If you are ever unsure of the safest practice, never hesitate to ask a professional. Remember to always listen to your body.

Physical activity around the world

Physical activity is promoted differently around the world. In 2018, The WHO (2018b) found that of the 28 countries in the European Union (EU), 21 countries, or 75%, had a national program to promote physical activity. While most countries had promotion techniques, it is important to remember that media and communication strategies alone are not effective in promoting behavior change. The EU encourages improving the promotion of physical activity in senior centers and in the workplace (WHO, 2018b). Examples of health promotion techniques that promote living a physically active life include advertisements and campaigns throughout various cities worldwide that encourage individuals to get up and get moving, such as scavenger hunts. Examples of these city scavenger hunts have been seen in Paris, France, Johannesburg, Gauteng, and Boston, Massachusetts (ScavengerHunt.com, 2019). Other examples seen globally are historical walking trails through cities and adult playgrounds.

In his own words

Austyn, 25. African American, male

I played lacrosse and tennis through high school but stopped playing when I entered college. It wasn't until a friend of mine invited me to join him in trying a free trial at a local rock-climbing gym that I really got back into working out. Looking back, I think I stopped playing sports because I missed the team environment and the challenge of the game. Getting into rock-climbing has begun to fill that gap. Our gym offers yoga, too, and I started about a year ago. Man, has that been life changing for my mental well-being! It's nice to challenge my mind and body in different ways. My one regret is that I didn't start sooner!

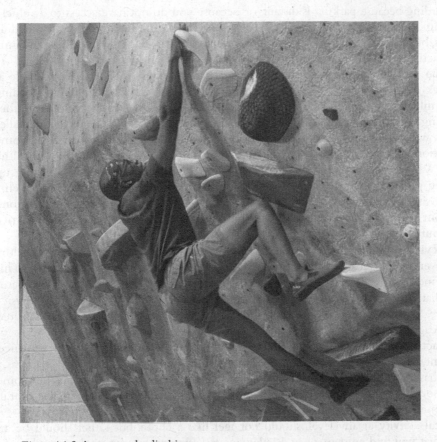

Figure 14.2 Austyn rock-climbing.
Source: This image was provided by Kayla K. McDonald.

Physical activity through the various phases of life

Physical activity looks different throughout various phases of life. As a child, physical activity is instilled in our daily activities – playing on the playground, going to physical education classes, walking to and from classes, and playing outside. As we age, our lives naturally become more sedentary, from sitting at a desk at work to your daily commute. Becoming more intentional about getting up and moving becomes more important in our daily lives.

Different types of exercise are more imperative in different phases of life. As we age, ensuring core stability and balance is important in preventing falls (Mayo Clinic, 2005). As we go through life, our bodies and abilities change, and it is important to recognize the role that plays on the range of mobility.

Throughout the many phases of life, the setting we are in changes, and that can impact what kind of physical activity we participate in. For example, college campuses are often set up differently than the town you may have grown up in or the town you may move to after this phase of your life. On a college campus you may see more walking, biking, and skateboarding because parking is distant, or because you do not have access to a vehicle. Attending a fitness class at the local gym may be challenging because of your schedule restraints, but you may walk across campus to meet your friends for lunch. While the time you are active is not necessarily structured, you are still staying active.

On the other hand, simple changes in your current environment may be possible as well. Let's consider an office setting. Perhaps your office provides adjustable standing or treadmill desks to encourage standing and moving throughout the workday, rather than sitting. Another strategy that is simpler, is encouraging walking meetings for smaller meetings with 1–3 people to encourage movement while still getting work done. Some organizations may even offer yoga at lunch time once a week to promote a healthy lifestyle. While some days it may seem stressful to get up and get moving, getting up and being physically active will help clear the mind and allow you to work more efficiently. Thinking outside of the box often helps in controlling the sedentary situations. Ask if your workplace has any worksite wellness programs to encourage you to be active throughout the day.

As previously mentioned, physical activity is an important part of living a healthy life for everyone, regardless of age, race, religion, among other social determinants. This includes individuals of varying abilities. Adapted, or modified, physical activity programs ensure that individuals of various backgrounds can work toward being more physically active. Some common programs include Special Olympics, Senior Citizen/Retired Sports Leagues, in addition to other community-based programs. Specific benefits of physical activity for individuals with disabilities include balancing muscles, independence, enjoyment, and managing secondary conditions, which are conditions that develop as a result of having another health issue, like nerve damage (Mayo Clinic, 2005). While some activities or exercise plans may be modified for an individual with a disability, the overall health benefits are beneficial to the individual.

Physical activity, at any level, should not feel like a chore, but rather should be an activity that you find enjoyment in. In elementary classrooms, some teachers implement dancing in between assignments/subjects. Some senior centers have used Wii bowling tournaments to encourage physical engagement among residents. Universities, like George Mason University, have promoted "Who's Walking Wednesday," a walking meeting, on their campus to promote walking while discussing campus initiatives with various staff and faculty (George Mason University, 2019). Your interests in various activities may vary throughout your lifetime but valuing your active time can have health benefits that are well worth the pay off. In many countries around the world, technology plays a large role in people's involvement with physical activity.

Technology's role in physical activity

Over many decades, the transition of hands-on work to sedentary work, in addition to the accessibility of media available online and through various platforms has been proven to displace some of the regular physical activity in the average life (Maibach, 2007). The accessibility of handheld technology today is suggested to have contributed to the decline in physical activity and the increase in related chronic diseases (Maibach, 2007). Compare the use of televisions today to the 1960s and 1970s. If you wanted to change the channel back then, you would have to get up from the sofa and turn the dial. Nowadays we have remotes that we can talk to and don't even need to lift a finger. The improvements in technology have reduced the physical activity that used to come with watching television, but there have been some advances related to other forms of physical activity that have come from technological innovation.

Recent technological advances have begun to play a large role in the realm of physical activity; from smart gym machines, to smart watches, there seems to be a nifty gadget to monitor everything possible. Not only do these electronic devices help to track the ups and downs of workouts, but they track how many steps one has taken, their heart rate, sleep patterns, plus they even buzz to remind you of prolonged inactivity. These activity trackers, such as Garmin watches, Fitbits, Apple watches, and others, serve as tools to encourage physical activity, as well as motivation, including challenges that you participate in with virtual peers.

Evolving technology has opened a new world colliding with physical activity through global positioning system role playing games (GPS RPGs) that get individuals up and moving, such as Pokémon Go and Orna. These games use the local geography and the main components of video games to get people out and moving to "Catch 'Em All" (Page, 2019). The idea of taking a sedentary activity and making it active can aid in addressing health concerns related to sedentary lifestyles, especially within the video gaming community. The Guardian (2016) explains that these apps are not marketed as health tools but are expected to have positive health effects.

More information

Physical activity is a necessary component to living a healthier and happier life, but it is important to fully understand the ins and outs of the many kinds of physical activity. Most local libraries provide a collection of books related to physical activity and men's health. Some of these books are written by physical therapists in the field, physicians, athletes, and researchers. Recommended readings include: *The Encyclopedia of Exercise Anatomy* by Liebman for understanding the biomechanics of our bodies and various training plans, in addition to the *Men's Health Concerns Sourcebook* edited by Sandra J. Judd, for a variety of information on topics related to men's health, including physical activity.

In addition to available readings, Men's Health (2015) listed the following podcasts as the five best fitness podcasts:

- The Tim Ferriss Show
- Food for Fitness
- Mark Bell's PowerCast
- Bulletproof Radio
- Get-Fit Guy

Other recommended podcasts include Move Forward by the American Physical Therapy Association, All About Fitness with Pete McCall, and The Men's Health Podcast, all of which can be found where you listen to podcasts. These resources provide insight, often brought to the listener from a male perspective, regarding physical activity and men's health.

Through social media, information on physical activity and the benefits can be found through following accounts such as The Centers for Disease Control and Prevention, The American Heart Association, The American Cancer Association, The American Council of Exercise, The World Health Organization, among others. Additional professional advice can be sought out through certified personal trainers, your primary care physician, and physical therapists.

Key next steps

In order to best understand the role that physical activity plays specifically in the life of a man, more specific research must be conducted. A large amount of the research on the topic, globally and in the United States, lacks information that separates physical activity data on gender. Individuals should continue to advocate for the physical activities that they enjoy, regardless of the stereotypes that are present, like with yoga. Understanding the effects of physical activity, and lack of physical activity, will assist in the community's understanding of why physical activity is beneficial specifically to men.

Conclusion

Physical activity involves movement of the body that increases the heart rate of a person (Mayo Clinic, 2005). While globally it is recommended that individuals participate in a minimum of 150 minutes of moderate physical activity each week, many individuals still don't reach this (WHO, 2018a). The result of living a life that is more sedentary than active is often related to increased risk of chronic diseases such as heart disease, obesity, type 2 diabetes and high blood pressure, among other conditions. Introducing physical activity and/or exercise into an individual's life should happen in incremental steps and begin by introducing minor lifestyle changes. By getting out and moving through a variety of activities, individuals are more likely to live a healthier and happier life.

Personal assessment

- Do you maintain a physically active life?
- What could you implement in your life to be more physically active?

References

American Heart Association. (2018). *American Heart Association recommendations for physical activity in adults and kids.* Retrieved from www.heart.org/en/healthy-living/fitness/fitness-basics/aha-recs-for-physical-activity-in-adults

Centers for Disease Control and Prevention. (2017). *Exercise or physical activity.* Retrieved from www.cdc.gov/nchs/fastats/exercise.htm

Centers for Disease Control and Prevention. (2019). *Walking.* Retrieved from www.cdc.gov/physicalactivity/walking/index.htm

Chertoff, J. (2018). *What's the difference between aerobic and anaerobic?* Retrieved from www.healthline.com/health/fitness-exercise/difference-between-aerobic-and-anaerobic

George Mason University. (2019). *Who's walking Wednesday with Frank Neville.* Retrieved from www2.gmu.edu/news/578141

The Guardian. (2016). *Pokémon Go can boost health by making gamers exercise, says GP.* Retrieved from www.theguardian.com/technology/2016/aug/10/pokemon-go-health-players-exercise-obesity-walking

Guthold, R., Stevens, G. A., Riley, L. M., & Bull, F. C. (2018). Worldwide trends in insufficient physical activity from 2001 to 2016: A pooled analysis of 358 population-based surveys with 1.9 million participants. *The Lancet: Global Health, 6*(10). Retrieved from www.thelancet.com/journals/langlo/article/PIIS2214-109X(18)30357-7/fulltext

Hales, D. (2017). *An Invitation to Health: The power of now.* Boston, MA: Cengage Learning.

Macmillan Support Group. (2016). *How active should I be?* Retrieved from www.macmillan.org. uk/information-and-support/bowel-cancer/rectal/coping/maintaining-a-healthy-lifestyle/ keeping-active/how-active-should-i-be.html

Maibach, E. (2007). The influence of the media environment on physical activity: Looking for the big picture. *American Journal of Health Promotion: AJHP, 21*(1), 353–362.

Mayo Clinic. (2005). *Fitness for Everybody.* Rochester, MN: Mayo Clinic Health Information.

Mayo Clinic. (2019). *6 compelling exercise benefits for men.* Retrieved from http://diet.mayoclinic. org/diet/move/exercise-benefits-for-men

Men's Health. (2015). *5 best fitness podcasts.* Retrieved from www.menshealth.com/uk/fitness/ a754817/5-best-fitness-podcasts/

Pacific Prime. (2013). *The top 5 most common men's sports injuries.* Retrieved from www.pacificprime. com/blog/the-top-5-most-common-mens-sports-injuries.html

Page, D. (2019). *The best GPS and location-based games on mobile.* Retrieved from www.pockettactics. com/guides/location-based-games-ios-android/

Prochaska, J. O., & Velicer, W. F. (1997). The transtheoretical model of health behavior change. *American Journal of Health Promotion: AJHP, 12*(1), 38–48. https://doi.org/10.4278/0890-1171-12.1.38

Remski, M. (2017). *10 things we didn't know about yoga until this new must-read dropped.* Retrieved from www.yogajournal.com/yoga-101/10-things-didnt-know-yoga-history

ScavengerHunt.com. (2019). *All our locations.* Retrieved from www.scavengerhunt.com/locations/ all_scavenger_hunts.php

Tilin, A. (2017). *Yoga for men: why you should be practicing.* Retrieved from www.yogajournal.com/ practice/man-factor

UCHealth. (2016). *Benefits of combining aerobic and anaerobic exercise into daily workouts.* Retrieved from https://medfit.org/benefits-combining-aerobic-anaerobic-exercise-daily-workouts/

World Health Organization. (2018a). *Physical activity.* Retrieved from www.who.int/news-room/ fact-sheets/detail/physical-activity

World Health Organization. (2018b). *Promoting physical activity in the health sector.* Retrieved from www.euro.who.int/__data/assets/pdf_file/0008/382337/fs-health-eng.pdf

Index

Printed in the United States
by Baker & Taylor Publisher Services